Pocket
On Call

Pocket
On Call

Andrew Stewart
Specialist Registrar in Anaesthetics and
Intensive Care Medicine
Sheffield, UK

Editorial advisor
Rory Mackinnon
GP Registrar
Newcastle, UK

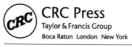

CRC Press
Taylor & Francis Group
Boca Raton London New York

CRC Press is an imprint of the
Taylor & Francis Group, an **informa** business

Cover image supplied by Dr Richard Dachtler, General Practitioner, Sheffield, UK.

CRC Press
Taylor & Francis Group
6000 Broken Sound Parkway NW, Suite 300
Boca Raton, FL 33487-2742

© 2015 by Andrew Stewart
CRC Press is an imprint of Taylor & Francis Group, an Informa business

No claim to original U.S. Government works

Printed on acid-free paper
Version Date: 20141204

International Standard Book Number-13: 978-1-4441-8503-4 (Paperback)

Library of Congress Cataloging-in-Publication Data

Stewart, Andrew, active 2014, author.
    Pocket on call / Andrew Stewart.
    p. ; cm. -- (Pocket series)
Includes bibliographical references and index.
    Summary: "The only pocket-sized guide dedicated to preparing for and being on call, Pocket On Call is ideal for use in the busy clinical setting convenient - everything the student or junior needs at their fingertips, portable - genuine pocket format, illustrated - clear, simple and reproducible explanatory line diagrams enhance the text, tailored - written specifically with the inexperienced doctor in mind, Answering the questions that you are too scared or embarrassed to ask, with this book as your indispensable companion, medical students and junior doctors will be equipped to tackle being on call appropriately and with confidence"--Provided by publisher.
    ISBN 978-1-4441-8503-4 (paperback : alk. paper)
    I. Title. II. Series: Pocket series (Boca Raton, Fla.)
    [DNLM: 1. Medical Staff, Hospital--Handbooks. 2. Clinical Competence--Handbooks. 3. Needs Assessment--Handbooks. WX 39]

RA971.35
362.11068'3--dc23   2014013458

Visit the Taylor & Francis Web site at
http://www.taylorandfrancis.com

and the CRC Press Web site at
http://www.crcpress.com

To Lis

It is a huge pleasure to be asked to write a foreword for the first edition of *Pocket On Call* by Dr Andrew Stewart.

I am sure that medical students today have many frustrations with medical school education, but when I remember back to my days as a 'House Officer', my biggest frustration was why I was not more prepared practically for life as a junior doctor. I was a diligent student, I had an immense amount of medical and surgical knowledge, had passed exams and OSCEs but somehow the practicalities of assessing and treating patients during a busy on-call shift had completely passed me by. It was a tough learning curve but I had a great sense of achievement when I was able to master the role and run an efficient 'post-take' ward round.

As a consultant anaesthetist, I have spent years teaching medical students and F1/F2 doctors in the recognition and management of seriously ill patients. The most frequent question I am asked is, *"What things should I have done before I called my Registrar?"* Therefore I am so pleased that the content in this book emphasizes the important role of the F1 in making sure that a thorough history and examination have been undertaken, that all relevant investigations have been performed and that the results are available for senior review.

The content in this book is very suitable for final-year medical students, Foundation Year doctors and also Advanced Nurse Practitioners (ANP). With its succinct style, comprehensive contents and practical advice, this book will have an important role both as an educational tool and also as an aide-memoire when on call.

Writing a book like this is not an easy task. It requires a great deal of knowledge, attention to detail and insight into the target audience. Dr Stewart is to be congratulated on a superb text and one that students, junior doctors and nursing colleagues will find an invaluable resource.

I wish this book every success and look forward to recommending it to others.

Dr Anil Hormis
Consultant in Anaesthesia, Critical Care
& Pre-hospital Emergency Medicine
Rotherham NHS Foundation Trust

Section A

'Getting set'

So you've made it! Finals already seem like a distant memory and you've even survived the 'trust induction'. Now the real fun starts!

Being on call as an F1 can be daunting. You find yourself roaming the empty corridors of a deserted hospital and you quickly discover that you are often the first port of call for acutely unwell patients across the hospital.

The aim of this handbook is to hopefully alleviate some of the stress from those first few on-call shifts. With each topic, the aim is to deliver a strategy for the immediate assessment and optimisation of the patient. In particular, the focus is centred on the management steps that would be appropriate for the new F1 doctor, with additional tips and hints that may not have been taught in the lecture theatre.

I hope you find this handbook useful.

Generally speaking, on-call responsibilities can be split into 'take' and 'cover'.

The 'take'

'Take' refers to new patients admitted to a particular speciality over a 24-hour period. So for example, 'medical take' are all the patients admitted to medicine. New patients are referred from two main sources; either directly from the emergency department (ED) or from GPs in the community (often known as 'bed bureau' admissions). Doctors taking part in the take are responsible for accepting the referral [usually the senior house officer (SHO) or specialist registrar (SPR)]* and for the clerking and initial management of the patient. Most hospitals now operate designated wards for the care of new patients admitted to the hospital, usually referred to as assessment units – medical or surgical assessment units, for example.

---

* Technically, in the UK at least, 'SHO' and 'SPR' no longer exist. They are old terms replaced with a multitude of new titles (including: FY2, CT1/2, ST1/2, Trust Doctor – this is just for the 'SHO' grade alone!). In reality however, hospitals still use SHO and SPR, as the new terms are confusing to many staff and often don't explain the seniority. Everyone knows what 'SHO' means but not necessarily 'Core Trainee Year 2'.

Ward cover

During the day, all wards are staffed by teams of doctors working for particular consultants. Between 5 p.m. and 8 or 9 a.m. the following morning, service provision is provided by a much smaller number of 'on-call' doctors whose job it is to provide medical or surgical cover across the hospital. The exact nature of the on-call team will vary between trusts and will depend on the size and activity level of the hospital, as well as the services which are provided. Overnight, some hospitals now run 'hospital at night' schemes whereby a coordinator (usually a senior sister or charge nurse) accepts bleeps from across the hospital and distributes the workload to the appropriate medical and surgical teams.

These tips may make things run a little more smoothly:

- Check your rota closely – they are not always easy to follow!
- Make sure you fully understand your on-call responsibilities before you start (i.e. which wards you are covering).
- Make a note of important bleeps, extensions and door codes: a cheat sheet sometimes helps.
- Ensure you have all the relevant passwords for your hospital's computers to allow access to blood results, x-rays, etc.
- Give yourself a test bleep when your shift begins – as appealing as a broken bleep may seem, you need to be contactable at all times.
- Food and drink are a must! Bring some with you or make sure you know where and when food is available at your hospital.
- Equipment: Some pieces of kit are vital; hunting for a tourniquet on an unfamiliar ward at 3 a.m. is no fun!
- Locate your nearest blood gas analyser and know how to use it.
- Familiarize yourself with your hospital's crash trolley and defibrillator before your first on call: resuscitation officers are usually happy to help with this.

Equipment checklist

- Stethoscope.
- Tourniquet.
- Bleep – checked and working.
- Pens – at least two, black ink only.
- Notebook – to write down important details as you go (i.e. patient details and location). As busy as you will be, taking a few seconds to make legible notes is well worth it.
- Food and drink.
- Watch – but not on your wrist.

Bleeps to note

Make a note of the following bleeps:

- Your team: SHO and SPR (senior house officer, specialist registrar).
- Radiographer.
- Blood bank.
- First on-call anaesthetist.
- Haematology, biochemistry, and microbiology lab numbers for results.
- Site manager.

Key points

- The 'take' refers to all new patients referred to hospital specialties in a given 24-hour period.
- Ward 'cover' is the provision of medical support to hospital wards out of hours.
- Take time to prepare for on-call work.
- Check your equipment before each shift.
- Note down important bleeps and extension numbers.

Section B

Acutely unwell patients

During on-call shifts, acutely unwell patients may be brought to your attention in a number of ways.

Handover: The structure of this will vary between hospitals. Typically, there will be a 'handover' from the day teams at the end of a normal working day. Any outstanding jobs or patients who have been particularly unwell during the day will be handed over to the on-call 'cover' team. This may be via an electronic computer-based system or by verbal communication.

Emergency buzzers: These are usually activated by pulling an ominous red button which can be found attached to the wall in most bed spaces. Their appearance will vary between hospitals, and it is worth familiarizing yourself with what they look (and sound) like in your hospital.

Cardiac arrest bleep: In most hospitals the cardiac arrest team consists of the on-call medical team, the on-call anaesthetist, and sometimes a senior nurse from the cardiac care unit (CCU) or the emergency department (ED). The bleep tone is usually faster and prolonged and is followed by a speech message alerting you to the location of the arrest.

Fast bleep: These pages are received when a doctor is required urgently and will usually sound similar to the cardiac arrest bleep.

Early warning scores: Most hospitals now operate early warning score (EWS) systems as a means of rapidly identifying deteriorating patients. Every time nursing staff record clinical observations (OBS) a total score is generated based on whether the numbers are within or stray outside of set physiological parameters. Abnormal observations will generate a number; the more abnormal the physiology, the higher the number. Depending on the score generated, the nursing staff will request a medical review within a designated time frame. The following illustrates an example of a typical early warning score.

The National Early Warning System (NEWS)

The NEWS system is a new early warning tool produced in collaboration with the Royal Colleges of Physicians and Nursing and the National Outreach Forum. It is set to become the gold standard across the country. The diagram on page 11, reprinted with permission from the Royal College of Physicians, displays the NEWS system as it would appear on the back of the observation chart.

'Doctor, the patient's NEWS is ...'

This is a very common bleep from nursing staff, particularly during on-call shifts and out of hours. Consider asking the following over the phone before setting off to assess the patient:

- Score break down: Ask for the individual observations (OBS) (gives you an idea of what you are going to).

- Ask about trends: What is the patient's usual blood pressure (BP), heart rate (HR), etc.
- Why is the patient in the hospital? Working diagnosis?
- Any specific symptoms? Chest pain, shortness of breath (SOB), palpitations, etc.
- Past medical history (PMHx).

> **Remember:** Depending on the situation, it may be possible to delegate certain tasks to nursing staff before you arrive (e.g. starting oxygen, repeating OBS); this can speed things up in an acute situation.

Physiological Parameters	3	2	1	0	1	2	3
Respiration Rate	≤8		9–11	12–20		21–24	≥25
Oxygen Saturations	≤91	92–93	94–95	≥96			
Any Supplemental Oxygen		Yes		No			
Temperature	≤35.0		35.1–36.0	36.1–38.0	38.1–39.0	≥39.1	
Systolic BP	≤90	91–100	101–110	111–219			≥220
Heart Rate	≤40		41–50	51–90	91–110	111–130	≥131
Level of Consciousness				A			V, P, or U

*The NEWS initiative flowed from the Royal College of Physicians' NEWSDIG, and was jointly developed and funded in collaboration with the Royal College of Physicians, Royal College of Nursing, National Outreach Forum and NHS Training for Innovation.

Royal College of Physicians

NHS
Training for Innovation

Rather conveniently, the first five letters of the alphabet also lay out the crucial five stages of the initial emergency assessment, or A, B, C, D, E examination. This is a well-established system used to rapidly examine and optimize any acutely unwell patient.

The basic principle is to assess each step in order, correcting any abnormality as soon as it is identified. Each and every patient you are called to see should receive an initial assessment using this systematic approach.

The basis of this is logical – in any acute situation, the overall emphasis is to ensure optimal oxygen delivery at the cellular level, in addition to correcting the underlying pathology. To achieve this you must have:

1. A patent, unobstructed airway (**A**).
2. Efficient gas exchange at the alveolar – capillary membrane (**B**).
3. An intact cardiovascular system to perfuse the lungs and carry oxygenated blood to tissues (**C**).

Step **D** stands for *disability*, and represents a focused neurological assessment.

Step **E** stands for *exposure* – a general top-to-toe assessment including factors such as body temperature, abdominal examination, and blood glucose measurement. (*Remember*:

Hypoglycaemia is a common cause of reduced Glasgow Coma Score (GCS) and is easily correctable.)

Your initial assessment will no doubt vary a little depending on the particular circumstances, but it is useful to consider the 'ideal' A, B, C, D, E assessment as a starting point.

The A, B, C, D, E assessment – in practice

It should be stressed this is different from the standard examination that accompanies a full medical clerking. The A, B, C, D, E approach is used in the context of the acutely unwell patient. The following provides a practical approach:

A – airway

Observe and speak to the patient: Is he or she maintaining his or her airway?

Optimize as appropriate using:

Airway manoeuvres – head tilt, chin lift, jaw thrust.

Airway adjuncts – oropharyngeal/nasal airway.

Suction of oropharynx if required.

B – breathing

Measure respiratory rate + assess breathing pattern.

Note position of trachea.

Auscultate the chest + expansion/resonance.

Attach pulse oximeter + consider arterial blood gas (ABG) if indicated.

Commence interventions as appropriate – oxygen, nebulizer, etc.

C – circulation

Pulse – assess rate, rhythm, and volume.
Measure BP.
Consider attaching heart monitor.
Central capillary refill time.
Auscultate praecordium.
Secure IV access + bloods + IV fluids as appropriate.
12-lead ECG if indicated.
If catheterized, measure urine output.

D – disability

Assess pupils.
Observe limb movement for reduced power/asymmetry.
GCS assessment.
Babinski/plantar reflex.

E – exposure

Measure core body temperature.
Abdominal examination.
Examine the calves for swelling, pain, asymmetry (think about deep vein thrombosis (DVT)).
Check glucose (don't forget the mantra 'never ever forget glucose').
Note any other stigmata of disease.

A note about the airway: Airway obstruction may be partial or complete and can occur both in patients with a low GCS (common) and in fully awake patients. Patients with a low GCS obstruct their airway due to a combination of reduced pharyngeal muscle tone ± vomit/secretions. Fully conscious patients may also develop airway obstruction, for example; patients with epiglottitis, head and neck tumours, goitres, foreign body inhalation, etc.

Key points

- Acutely unwell patients may be brought to your attention via an EWS system, handover, fast bleeps or cardiac arrest calls.
- The NEWS system is a standardized early warning system used increasingly across hospital trusts.
- Utilize the A, B, C, D, E assessment for each and every acutely unwell patient you are called to review.

You will frequently be asked to review patients complaining of chest pain. As a symptom, chest pain may originate from any structure within the chest wall, thoracic cavity, or mediastinum.

As a result, the potential causes are numerous and range from the trivial to the immediately life threatening. In reality, the main concern with chest pain is that it may represent life-threatening pathology, most commonly:

- Acute coronary syndromes (ACS). The umbrella term for ST segment elevation myocardial infarction (STEMI), non-ST segment elevation myocardial infarction (NSTEMI), or unstable angina (UA).
- Pulmonary embolus (PE).

Rarer life-threatening causes to keep in mind include tension pneumothorax and thoracic aortic dissection.

Focused assessment

In addition to the initial A, B, C, D, E assessment, consider the following for all patients with chest pain:

- Take a history regarding the characteristics of the pain. This will help you formulate an appropriate differential diagnosis list.
- Full set of clinical observations.
- 12-lead ECG. (Arrange for *all* patients. PE and MI can both demonstrate characteristic ECG changes.)

- Chest auscultation/assessment. (May indicate a primary pulmonary cause, and acute MI can cause secondary left ventricular failure.)
- Cardiovascular exam. (MI may cause acute ventricular septal defect (VSD) or mitral valve prolapse. Both can cause a systolic murmur. Pulse assessment may reveal tachycardia or arrhythmia. Jugular venous pressure (JVP) is often difficult to assess, but if markedly elevated, it may indicate large PE or right ventricular infarct.)
- Chest wall palpation. Reproducibility on palpation may indicate musculoskeletal origin but does not rule out an additional, more serious cause.
- Blood pressure measurement for both arms. Significant inequality between readings may suggest thoracic aortic dissection.
- Analgesia. Address this early – this is as important to the patient as treating the cause!
- Senior review. Particularly when starting out, it is worth discussing all patients with chest pain with a senior.

Chest pain: common presentations and management

Pulmonary embolism

- **Presentation:** Highly variable. Dependent on size and position of embolus within the pulmonary arterial tree. Symptoms are usually acute onset, but not always. Chest pain is usually pleuritic (due to infarction of adjacent parietal pleura) or similar to typical MI pain (due to distension of the pulmonary artery proximal to a large embolus). Also look for SOB + tachypnoea (can be the only presenting feature), sometimes cough or haemoptysis is also present. A large PE may cause cardiovascular collapse or cardiac arrest.

- **Risk factors:** Anything that reduces blood flow in a large vein: immobility, lower limb surgery, pelvic pathology, or factors promoting a pro-thrombotic state: active cancer, combined oral contraceptive pill, dehydration, clotting disorders (e.g. factor V Leiden deficiency).
- **Investigations:**
  - ECG: May reveal nothing of note. The most common finding is simply sinus tachycardia. With a large PE, look for right bundle branch block (RBBB) and right-axis deviation.
  - Plain chest radiograph (chest x-ray; CXR): The lung fields are usually clear (i.e. the CXR is usually normal).
  - CTPA (CT pulmonary angiogram): The gold standard for diagnosis, but is usually undertaken after treatment has commenced.
- **Treatment:** Supplemental oxygen to correct hypoxaemia + secure intravenous access. Provide a therapeutic dose of a low molecular weight heparin (LMWH) given as a subcutaneous injection (the exact drug available will vary between trusts; therefore, follow local protocols). If there is marked cardiovascular instability, then thrombolysis is usually considered. Typically this involves an intravenous bolus of a thrombolytic agent (e.g. alteplase) followed by an infusion over the next 24 hours.

The new F1: If you suspect a PE, call for senior help early. In this context you will usually not be expected to begin treatment yourself, but consider doing the following:

- Start appropriate oxygen therapy (see later section).
- Send bloods: Full blood count (FBC), urea and electrolytes (U&E), clotting screen (CLS) (and label as urgent).
- ECG + portable CXR.
- Arterial blood gas (ABG).

Remember: PE can be a difficult diagnosis, and a low index of suspicion is required. With typical symptoms, risk factors, and no focal chest signs/clear CXR, think PE until proven otherwise.

Acute coronary syndrome

- **Presentation:** Typically, central or left anterior chest pain with or without radiation to left arm, neck, or jaw. Described as pressure, heaviness, or aching sensation. Look for associated nausea and vomiting, pallor, and SOB (sometimes due to secondary left ventricular failure, but may occur in association with isolated myocardial ischaemia).
- **Risk factors:** Pre-existing ischaemic heart disease (IHD), smoking, diabetes mellitus, high cholesterol, strong family history, hypertension.
- **Investigation:** ´
  - 12-lead ECG: Typical changes are ST segment elevation or new LBBB (both of which indicate transmural infarction). ST depression and T-wave

inversion are associated with NSTEMI or unstable angina. Arrhythmias or conduction defects may also be seen. *Note*: Where possible, always compare with previous ECGs to help establish whether changes are new or old.

- **Treatment:** Each hospital will have set guidelines for the management of acute coronary syndromes which are worth studying before you start on-call shifts. The following would be typical:
  - Aspirin 300mg PO.
  - Clopidogrel 300mg PO [usually 600mg if STEMI going for percutaneous coronary intervention (PCI)]. (Note: Some trusts now use ticagrelor instead of clopidogrel.)
  - Morphine 1–10mg IV + anti-emetic.
  - Glyceryl trinitrate (GTN): Either spray or buccal.
  - Low molecular weight heparin as a subcutaneous injection [or IV if going for PCI].
  - Supplemental oxygen as appropriate to correct hypoxaemia (if present).
- All patients with acute MI should ideally be allocated to a monitored bed.

Remember: Morphine, oxygen, nitrate, aspirin, clopidogrel (MONAC).

Additional causes for chest pain

As noted in the introduction to this chapter, chest pain may reflect pathology arising from any organ or structure within the thoracic cavity, mediastinum or chest wall. Whilst the initial focus should be to investigate for the presence of ACS or PE (as these are common and potentially life threatening) it is important to consider other potential causes when assessing patients with chest pain.

Gastro-oesophageal reflux disease (GORD)

This is a common disorder resulting from dysfunction of the lower oesophageal sphincter, giving rise to symptoms that can be similar in nature to ACS. Typically, patients describe an intermittent, retrosternal 'burning' sensation that is sometimes relieved by sitting forwards. Patients may experience acid in the back of their mouths and often relate symptoms to particular types of food. Those at particular risk include the obese population and patients with a hiatus hernia.

Aortic dissection

Aortic dissections classically give rise to central burning/tearing chest pain that is sudden in onset and radiates through to the patient's back. Patients usually have either hypertension or a connective tissue disorder (e.g. Marfan's syndrome). Whilst several classification systems exist, aortic dissections are most often classified as either type A (involving the ascending aorta) or type B (not involving the ascending aorta). Type A dissections require urgent surgical intervention whilst type B dissections are managed medically.

Chest pain of musculoskeletal origin

Chest pain may arise from any type of tissue within the chest wall. Typically the pain is localized, worse on movement and is reproducible on palpation. However, be vigilant, reproducibility does not fully exclude an alternative cause for the chest pain. Diagnoses to consider include: rib fractures, muscular injury, costochondritis (idiopathic inflammation of the costochondral joint) and occasionally metastatic deposits.

Pleuritic causes

Pathology involving the lungs can give rise to so-called 'pleuritic' chest pain via inflammation of the adjacent parietal pleura. Common causes include pneumonia, peripheral PE, lung malignancy and pneumothorax. Rarer causes to keep in mind include rheumatoid disease, sarcoidosis and SLE (systemic lupus erythematosis) – all of which can produce deposits or inflammation affecting the parietal pleura.

Acute causes of chest pain

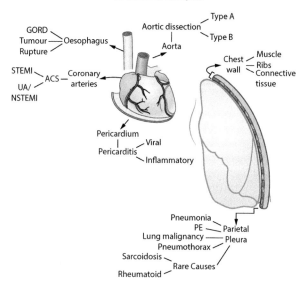

Key points

- Chest pain may represent a wide range of underlying disease processes.
- Consider the diagnosis of ACS and PE for every patient complaining of chest pain.
- Perform a 12-lead ECG for all patients in this group.
- Provide analgesia in addition to treating the pathology.

Shortness of breath (SOB) is a symptom common to all acute respiratory disorders and encompasses a wide spectrum, from patients who are 'a little' out of breath to patients who are significantly unwell requiring immediate treatment. A basic approach to the patient should include:

1. Observation from the end of the bed to assess work of breathing and general condition. (Essentially, how sick does the patient look?)
2. Focused history and respiratory examination.
3. Investigations.
4. Identification of the underlying cause.
5. Specific treatment for the disorder, appropriate use of supplemental oxygen, and supportive therapy.

Observation

Simple observation from the end of the bed is arguably the best indicator of how unwell the patient is. Look for:

- Speech: Can the patient talk in full sentences? Broken sentences? Single words?
- Respiratory rate.
- Use of accessory muscles.
- Fixing of shoulder girdles.
- Grunting.
- Cyanosis.

History

The quality of the history will obviously vary depending on how able the patient is to communicate. Also, talk to ward staff and look in the patient's notes. Consider the following:

- Onset (acute/gradual) and duration of SOB.
- Any similar episodes previously?
- Presence of associated symptoms – cough, sputum, chest pain, haemoptysis.
- Pre-existing respiratory problems (or those that may cause SOB, e.g. CCF).
- Reason for admission to hospital – always important to know. Does the patient already have a respiratory diagnosis – chronic obstructive pulmonary disease (COPD) exacerbation, pneumonia, etc.?
- OBS – look for trends, particularly SpO_2. Any recent blood gas results?
- Past medical history.

Examination

This should consist of the standard respiratory examination with an emphasis on chest auscultation (usually considered more beneficial in the acute setting than percussion, etc.). Where possible, check the initial clerking to ascertain whether chest signs you find are new or old. The following interpretation of chest signs is a very superficial guide, but may quickly get you into the ball park in an emergency:

- New, unilateral crackles or bronchial breathing – think pneumonia.

- Bilateral crackles – consider pulmonary oedema; either cardiogenic or acute respiratory distress syndrome (ARDS).
- Unilateral reduced breath sounds – pneumothorax, pleural effusion or atelectasis/lobe collapse.
- High-pitch wheeze – asthma, COPD, anaphylaxis, pulmonary oedema.

Investigations

In the initial phase of a respiratory emergency only a small number of investigations need to be considered:

- Plain chest radiograph (portable if the patient is particularly unwell).
- ECG.
- ABG.
- Bloods: FBC, U&E, liver function test (LFT), clotting screen.

When to do an arterial blood gas (ABG): Whilst there are no hard-and-fast rules, ABGs form an important initial investigation for many patients who are acutely unwell. From a respiratory point of view, consider an ABG in the presence of:

- Acute respiratory distress from whatever cause, particularly with significant desaturation.
- Very high respiratory rate or drop in conscious level.

Causes to consider

Immediate diagnostic clarity may be easier said than done in the presence of a complex patient who is struggling to breathe, but the following are amongst the most common you are likely to see:

- COPD exacerbation.
- Pneumonia.
- Asthma exacerbation.
- Acute left ventricular failure (LVF) causing pulmonary oedema.
- Acute respiratory distress syndrome (ARDS).
- Pneumothorax.
- Anaphylaxis.
- Exacerbations of other respiratory disorders (e.g. bronchiectasis or cystic fibrosis).

> **Remember:** Assessing this group of patients may vary significantly depending on whether or not there is a diagnosis in place. For example, you may be called to see a breathless, hypoxic patient on a surgical ward who has recently undergone surgery, or a patient with a known COPD exacerbation who is becoming increasingly breathless.

Treatment of acute respiratory disorders

This can be considered in three parts:

1. Keep the patient sat up as much as possible.
2. Supplemental oxygen to correct hypoxaemia (see below).
3. Specific treatment for each disorder.

The following outlines the core specific treatments for the more common disorders.

Exacerbation of asthma

- Oxygen-driven nebulizer: Salbutamol (2.5–5mg) repeated as necessary.
- Steroids: Prednisolone 40mg orally once daily – usually continued for 5 days. Alternatively, hydrocortisone 100mg IV may be given if the patient is too breathless to swallow.
- Antibiotics: If history or bloods suggest infective precipitant.
- Maintenance fluids.
- Magnesium sulphate (1.2–2g): Give as an intravenous infusion (IVI) over 20 minutes. (This is an advanced intervention – on senior advice only.)

> **Beware:** Patients with acute asthma may deteriorate rapidly. Inform a senior at an early stage. Establish if the patient has previously required admission to the intensive care unit (ICU)/high dependency unit (HDU) and observe closely.

Pneumonia

- Take blood ± sputum cultures if expectorating.
- Intravenous antibiotics – determined by local hospital policy (you will usually receive a laminated card on your trust induction).
- Intravenous fluid – resuscitate as necessary if the patient has the systemic inflammatory response syndrome (SIRS).

Anaphylaxis

- Adrenaline: 0.5mg (1 in 1000) IM. Give into the deltoid or lateral thigh.
- Hydrocortisone 200mg IV.
- Chlorphenamine 10mg IV.
- Nebulized salbutamol (if evidence of wheeze).
- IV fluid resuscitation (avoid gelatin or starch-based fluid due to risk of cross-reaction – usually anaphalactoid).

Anaphylaxis is often dramatic and always life threatening – get help early!

Acute LVF causing pulmonary oedema

- Nitrate – initially GTN spray or a buccal preparation (although avoid if hypotensive).
- Loop diuretic – furosemide 40–80mg as an IV bolus.
- Diamorphine (on senior advice only).
- GTN infusion (as part of ongoing management following senior review).

> **Beware:** Patients who develop acute LVF develop pulmonary oedema, but may also become hypotensive – both being secondary to an impaired left ventricle. In the presence of impaired organ perfusion this would then be classified as cardiogenic shock. All of the above treatments may potentially cause hypotension, so exercise caution in this patient group and seek senior advice immediately.

COPD exacerbation

- Nebulized salbutamol (2.5–5mg) via *air*-driven nebulizer. Repeat as necessary. (Can add ipratropium 500µg via nebulizer.)
- Prednisolone 30mg orally once daily, usually for 7 days.
- Antibiotics: If history or bloods suggest infective cause (again, as for asthma).
- Aminophylline (usually a late option – seek senior guidance before starting this).
- Send sputum cultures where possible.

Many patients with an exacerbation of COPD develop type 2 respiratory failure. If initial medical management fails, BiPAP™ is usually commenced (see separate section).

Oxygen therapy

Oxygen therapy is used to treat hypoxaemia, which is assessed clinically using a pulse oximeter. The management of the hypoxaemic patient is essentially threefold:

1. Where possible, establish and treat the cause (as above).
2. Restore acceptable oxygen saturations using supplemental oxygen.
3. Monitor progress and adjust oxygen/treatment accordingly.

For any patient requiring oxygen, the two main questions are:

- **What target saturations should be aimed for?**
- **Which oxygen delivery device should be used?**

Target saturations

Does the patient have, or is at risk of suffering from chronic type 2 respiratory failure?

1. If the answer is yes, aim for saturations between 88 and 92%.
2. For all other patients, aim for saturations between 94 and 98%.

This is based on the British Thoracic Society (BTS) guidance on oxygen therapy.

Which patients fall into group 1?

Patients for whom target saturations should be set between 88 and 92% are those with *chronic type 2 respiratory failure* from whatever cause. Typically this includes moderate to severe COPD, chest wall deformity, kyphoscoliosos, and morbid obesity. The combination of raised pCO_2 and elevated bicarbonate demonstrated on arterial blood gas indicates a chronic type 2 picture.

Why do the targets differ?

This is a controversial area, but the following is generally agreed upon: by definition, patients with chronic type 2 respiratory failure have a chronically elevated pCO_2. As such, they can no longer utilize pCO_2 variation as the main stimulus for breathing, and instead rely on the arterial oxygen partial pressure. Therefore, it is theoretically possible that giving these patients 'too much' oxygen will depress their respiratory drive. However, it should be emphasized that this is a rare phenomenon, and all acutely unwell patients should receive high-flow oxygen in the resuscitation phase of their care. The British Thoracic Society (BTS) guideline for oxygen therapy provides comprehensive guidance and is considered the gold standard – they are available to all healthcare professionals and are well worth a read before commencing on-call work.

Oxygen delivery devices

A wide variety of oxygen delivery devices are commercially available, but fortunately only a small number will be commonly encountered in the general ward environment. Devices are described as either fixed performance (providing a fixed, predictable concentration of oxygen) or variable performance (where the oxygen delivered fluctuates depending on the patient's respiratory pattern as well as the flow of oxygen.) The following are common examples that you are likely to use on a regular basis:

Nasal cannulae:

- Variable performance device.
- Typical FiO_2: 28–36%.
- Flow rate: 2–4L/minute.
- Appropriate for patients requiring prolonged periods of oxygen therapy at low concentrations (e.g. stable COPD, chronic lung conditions, etc.).
- Generally comfortable for patients – allows eating, speaking, etc.

Venturi facemask (very useful!):

- Fixed performance device.

- Exact FiO_2 determined by the valve used (e.g. 24, 28, 35, 40, and 60% are all available).
- Flow rate: Required rate is printed on each valve and varies depending on FiO_2.
- System consists of a facemask with a venturi valve attachment, through which a fixed FiO_2 is provided.
- Useful in any situation where a fixed concentration of oxygen is required (e.g. COPD exacerbations). Also of use in any acute respiratory setting to rationalize a patient's oxygen requirement.

Hudson facemask:

- Variable performance.
- Typical FiO_2: 35–40%.
- Flow rate: 4–6L/minute.
- Used in theatre in the immediate post-operative period but seldom used elsewhere.

Reservoir mask:

- Variable performance.
- Typical FiO_2: 80% (with good seal).
- Essentially a Hudson mask with reservoir attachment to provide increased FiO_2.
- Flow rate: 10–15L/minute.
- Used for emergency situations requiring oxygen: e.g. peri-arrest patient, severe hypoxia.
- Tip: Place finger over valve to allow reservoir bag to fully inflate before use.

Respiratory support

When medical therapy and supplemental oxygen fail to treat the underlying respiratory problem, patients are often escalated to a critical care environment where different forms of respiratory support may be used. In some hospitals, non-invasive respiratory support is available on designated wards outside of critical care. Whilst it is beyond the scope of this book to discuss this topic in detail, a basic understanding of the key concepts is useful.

In a nutshell:

- CPAP: Used to treat type 1 respiratory failure (oxygenation problem)
- BiPAP: Used to treat type 2 respiratory failure (ventilation problem)

Both of the above are delivered via a tightly fitting facemask (although CPAP may also be administered through a hood device). In this context, they are termed 'non-invasive', implying that they are delivered through a facemask rather than an endotracheal tube.

CPAP

As the name suggests, CPAP provides a continuous positive airway pressure throughout the respiratory cycle, offering the most benefit during expiration. The starting pressure is usually 5cm H_2O, although this can be increased as necessary. CPAP improves oxygenation and is thus a treatment for type 1 respiratory failure.

CPAP improves functional residual capacity and recruits alveoli – both of which improve oxygenation. It also helps to reduce the patient's work of breathing, thus reducing the likelihood of the patient requiring intubation and mechanical ventilation. It also provides oxygen through a securely fitting facemask, so one can be confident that the patient is receiving the set FiO_2.

BiPAP

BiPAP provides two levels of pressure – a high pressure during inspiration (inspiratory positive airway pressure (IPAP)) and a low pressure on expiration (expiratory positive airway pressure (EPAP)). The high pressure delivered with the patient's inspiratory breath improves ventilation by increasing alveolar ventilation; this improves clearance of carbon dioxide and thus treats type 2 respiratory failure. Typical starting settings would be IPAP 15 and EPAP 5, titrated as required for the individual patient. BiPAP is most commonly used to treat patients with exacerbations of COPD, but is of benefit to any patient with a type 2 respiratory failure refractory to medical therapy.

Key points

- Observation from the end of the bed is a good marker of the extent of patient compromise.
- Treat hypoxaemia with supplemental oxygen via a suitable delivery device.
- Determine a suitable target SpO_2 for each patient and document this.
- Initiate specific treatments for the given working diagnosis.
- Consider whether or not arterial blood gas analysis is indicated.
- For patients failing to improve, advanced respiratory support may be indicated.

Upper gastrointestinal (GI) bleeds carry an overall 10% mortality and patients may decompensate rapidly. Typical presenting features are haematemesis, melaena, or a combination of the two. Whilst numerous potential causes exist, the two most common are peptic ulcer disease and oesophagogastric varices. In addition, beware patients taking nonsteroidal anti-inflammatory drugs (NSAIDs) or anticoagulants – both result in an increased risk of upper GI bleeding.

The essence of management is to promptly assess patients to determine whether or not the patient is haemodynamically unstable. The latter group requires immediate resuscitation followed by intervention to arrest the bleeding. This is usually an oesophagogastroduodenoscopy (OGD) in the first instance, but sometimes surgery or interventional radiology may be necessary.

As an F1, you may be asked to clerk a patient on the admissions unit or to review a patient who has had a bleeding episode on the ward. Make a senior aware at an early stage: these patients can rapidly deteriorate!

Basic management steps

In addition to the basic A, B, C, D, E assessment, consider the following for all patients with an acute bleed:

- **Ask yourself:** Is the patient haemodynamically *stable* or *unstable*? Assess using the usual parameters: HR, BP, capillary refill time (CRT), pallor, urine output, and conscious level. If the patient is shocked, request the presence of a senior doctor as a priority. The patient is likely to require urgent blood products and therapeutic intervention to stop the bleeding.
- **Inspect for quantity of blood loss/melaena:** Look at bed sheets, kidney dishes and ask nursing staff.
- **Give high-flow oxygen** if the patient is peri-arrest.
- **Secure IV access:** Ideally 2 wide-bore cannulae.
- **Positioning in bed:** If the patient is shocked, ideally place him or her in the left lateral position with head down tilt (if the bed has the ability to do so).
- **Take bloods:** FBC, U&E, clotting, LFT, and make sure a group and save or cross-match is sent. If the bleeding is catastrophic, then blood products are urgently required.
- **Consider the cause for the bleeding:** History, examination, clinical notes, drug Kardex. Any stigmata of liver disease? Pre-existing disease? Anticoagulants? NSAIDs?

Oesophagogastric varices

Consider as a likely cause in the presence of any stigmata of liver disease: jaundice, ascites, dilated superficial abdominal veins, hepatomegaly, etc. In addition to the basic management steps, consider the following:

1. **IV antibiotics:** Patients in this demographic are often immunocompromised. Up-to-date guidance from the National Institute of Clinical Excellence (NICE) is to offer prophylactic therapy.
2. **Terlipressin:** This reduces portal venous pressure and thus reduces active bleeding. In this context it is given as an IV bolus. Seek senior advice before administration.

Peptic ulcer disease

Suspect peptic ulcer disease (PUD) with an upper GI bleed associated with epigastric pain, previous history of gastritis/ulceration, or recent treatment with NSAIDs. Commence treatment as follows:

> **IV proton pump inhibitor (PPI):** Consider for all patients in this category, some units prefer PPIs to be commenced following OGD. Increasing gastric pH will stabilize blood clots, thus reducing further bleeding. The drug of choice is usually pantoprazole delivered either as a regular bolus dose or as a continuous intravenous infusion. Therapy is usually continued for several days post-endoscopy.

Risk assessment scores

Two main assessment scores exist for upper GI bleeds – the Rockall and Blatchford scores. These help to predict morbidity and mortality and also the risk of rebleeding. It is beyond the scope of this book to discuss these in depth, but a basic understanding of their use is important.

**Specific treatments to consider for the patient
with upper GI haemorrhage**

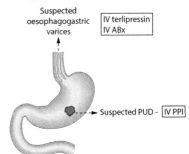

Suspected
oesophagogastric
varices

IV terlipressin
IV ABx

Discontinue →
• NSAIDS
• Oral anticoagulants
in both patient groups
following senior review

Suspected PUD - IV PPI

Key points

- Upper GI bleeds are common and potentially catastrophic.
- Oesophagogastric varices and PUD are the two most common causes.
- Determine whether or not the patient is cardiovascularly stable or unstable – this will alter the timing of endoscopic intervention.
- Consider terlipressin and antibiotics if varices are suspected.
- Consider PPI therapy for patients with likely PUD.

When clinicians refer to an acutely 'collapsed' patient, they are usually describing a patient who has suddenly lost consciousness, often in a dramatic fashion, either by falling to the floor or by collapsing backwards in bed. The altered consciousness level may be transient or sustained.

The potential causes are numerous, but can be quickly narrowed down by applying logic and basic principles. The crucial steps are to carry out a full A, B, C, D, E assessment and to gain a history from witnesses and nursing staff.

During the initial assessment process, consider the following:

Collateral history from nursing staff:

- What exactly happened? Ask any witnesses to describe what they saw.
- Any preceding symptoms? Chest pain, SOB, headache, etc.
- Reason for admission? Any recent changes to management? New drugs, etc.?
- Past medical history – check the notes if available.

For patients with a persisting low consciousness level, ask yourself the following to narrow down the potential causes:

- *Is the blood pressure acutely low compared to baseline observations?* If so, the collapse is likely due to reduced cerebral perfusion resulting from shock:

- **Cardiogenic:** Any chest pain? Palpitations? ECG abnormality? Arrhythmia?
- **Anaphylaxis:** Any new drugs or fluid given in the last few minutes? Rash? Pruritis? Known allergies? New wheeze? Stridor?
- **Sepsis:** Ongoing treatment for infection? New infective process? Pyrexia? Raised inflammatory markers?
- **Neurogenic:** Worth considering, but unlikely in the context of an acute collapse.
- **Hypovolaemic:** Visible blood loss? Recent surgery? Falling Hb? Known AAA?

- *Is the blood pressure normal?* In this situation, we can be confident that cerebral perfusion is adequate and shock is unlikely. Consider the following:

  - **Hypoglycaemia:** Diabetic history? Addison's disease? (Note – may also cause low BP.) Check glucose as a priority.
  - **Fitting/post-ictal:** Do witness accounts suggest a seizure? Check tongue for bite marks. Any incontinence?
  - **Cerebrovascular accident (CVA):** Check pupils for asymmetry/poor reactivity. Plantar reflex? Previous CVA/TIA? Abnormal limb movement? Hemiparesis?
  - **Head injury:** Any objective evidence of head injury? Suggestive history?
  - **Hypercapnia:** Raised $PaCO_2$ may be the cause of reduced consciousness (for example, severe type 2 respiratory failure) or may reflect a separate

pathology with secondary effects on respiratory system control due to pressure on the brain stem (e.g. CVA or head injury).

Patients with a transient loss of consciousness may have suffered an episode of syncope. Syncope is defined as a transient loss of consciousness secondary to cerebral hypoperfusion, which is followed by a rapid recovery. There are many different subtypes, and a careful history is required to reach a firm diagnosis. *Vasovagal syncope* is the 'simple' faint and represents a complex autonomic reflex. Patients experience a varied prodrome with features such as feeling hot and dizzy with wobbly legs. Patients make a rapid recovery following loss of consciousness. Other potential causes for transient loss of consciousness include concussion and short runs of significant cardiac dysrhythmias e.g. ventricular tachycardia.

Points to note: Neurogenic cardiac injury

Whilst most cases of persisting acute collapse with low BP are the result of shock, there is one notable exception. Following an acute intra-cranial event, various cardiovascular side effects may occur, many of which can result in low BP. This, therefore, provides a rare example whereby the patient's low level of consciousness may not be completely attributed to the co-existing hypotension.

The acutely collapsed patient — narrowing down the differentials

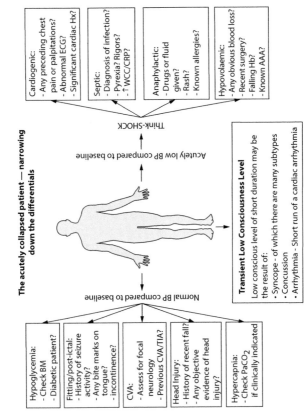

Think-SHOCK

Acutely low BP compared to baseline

Cardiogenic:
- Any preceding chest pain or palpitations?
- Abnormal ECG?
- Significant cardiac Hx?

Septic:
- Diagnosis of infection?
- Pyrexia? Rigors?
- ↑WCC/CRP?

Anaphylactic:
- Drugs or fluid given?
- Rash?
- Known allergies?

Hypovolaemic:
- Any obvious blood loss?
- Recent surgery?
- Falling Hb?
- Known AAA?

Normal BP compared to baseline

Hypoglycemia:
- Check BM
- Diabetic patient?

Fitting/post-ictal:
- History of seizure activity?
- Any bite marks on tongue?
- incontinence?

CVA:
- Assess for focal neurology
- Previous CVA/TIA?

Head Injury:
- History of recent fall?
- Any objective evidence of head injury?

Hypercapnia:
- Check PaCO2 if clinically indicated

Transient Low Consciousness Level

Low conscious level of short duration may be the result of:
- Syncope - of which there are many subtypes
- Concussion
- Arrhythmia - Short run of a cardiac arrhythmia

Key points

- Carry out a full and thorough A, B, C, D, E assessment and take a collateral history from nursing staff.
- Narrow down the differentials based on the patient's blood pressure.
- Acute, persisting low consciousness with associated low blood pressure is almost always due to a form of shock (septic, cardiogenic, anaphylactic, hypovolaemic etc.)
- Record blood glucose for each and every patient with an acute collapse.

Whilst many different types of seizure exist, when staff in hospital refer to a 'fitting patient', they are generally making reference to a 'tonic clonic' seizure. These manifest as a loss of consciousness with repeated and often vigorous motor movements of all four limbs. Being faced with a fitting patient can be quite alarming at first, but fortunately the basic management steps are logical and straightforward.

Management can be considered in two parts:

1. Steps taken to optimize the patient and stop the seizure.
2. History, examination and investigations to identify the underlying cause.

Optimizing the patient and seizure termination

- **Position:** Ideally place the patient in the left lateral position. This may be difficult if the patient is very large or the seizure is particularly vigorous. Protect the patient from hard objects and surfaces with pillows or blankets.
- **Oxygen:** Give high-flow oxygen at 15L/minute via a reservoir mask.
- **Airway:** Fitting patients often clench their teeth and many will hypersalivate. A nasopharyngeal (NP) airway is the adjunct of choice if the airway is obstructed, accompanied by suction. (Exercise caution when using the NP airway if a head injury is suspected – see below.)

- **IV access:** Secure at least one point of wide-bore IV access.
- **Timing:** Start the clock. Ask a nurse or staff member to time the seizure using a clock or stopwatch. It is generally agreed that drugs should be given to terminate a fit when the duration has reached 5 minutes.
- **Drugs:** The first-line drug for a tonic clonic seizure is a benzodiazepine – **intravenous lorazepam 4mg as a slow bolus over 1 to 2 minutes** is most commonly used. A further 4mg may be given if the initial bolus fails. Benzodiazepines can cause respiratory arrest – ensure you have a resus trolley immediately available. If the seizure continues, the next stage is to commence a **phenytoin infusion with a loading dose of 15–20mg/kg.** Failing this, the patient is given a full general anaesthetic.

Note: If alcohol withdrawal is strongly suspected as the underlying cause, then phenytoin is not indicated.

Caution: Beware using NP airways in patients with head injury. If a patient has an anterior basal skull fracture, there is a theoretical risk that the NP airway may pass through the sphenoidal sinus into the brain. Therefore, if a NP airway is the only immediate option available in a patient with a head injury and an obstructed airway, the decision should be made by a senior doctor.

Establishing the cause

Patients can fit for a wide variety of reasons. Common causes to consider are:

1. Epilepsy/seizure disorder.
2. Alcohol withdrawal.
3. Hypoglycaemia. (Always measure blood glucose as a priority in any fitting patient.)
4. Intracranial haemorrhage.
5. Hypoxia.
6. Head injury.
7. Overdose.
8. Fever.
9. Central nervous system (CNS) infection.

This is by no means a complete list but reflects the more common causes you are likely to come across.

The causes can usually be narrowed down effectively by taking a history from nursing staff, looking through the patient's notes and drug card, and examining the patient.

> **Remember:** Hypoglycaemia is a very reversible cause of fitting – make sure that glucose is measured during the resuscitation phase. This is very easy to forget amidst the organized chaos of a resuscitation effort.

Investigations

Common investigations typically include:

- Bloods – FBC, U&E, clotting (CLS), blood glucose ± blood cultures if pyrexial.
- Glucose.
- CT head.
- ABG.

Summary of immediate management

- High-flow oxygen.
- Left lateral position.
- Consider NP airway.
- IV access.
- Lorazepam 4mg IV bolus.
- Glucose measurement.

Key points

- Tonic clonic seizures are the most common in general hospital practice.
- Take steps both to optimize the patient and to diagnose the underlying cause.
- A nasopharyngeal airway is the initial adjunct of choice for airway support during a seizure.
- Drugs are given once the patient has been fitting for 5 minutes.
- The initial agent used is typically lorazepam, 4mg as a slow IV bolus.

Acute abdominal pain is a very common presentation with a wide range of potential causes. In the majority of cases, abdominal pain reflects pathology involving intra-abdominal or pelvic organs, but the abdominal wall and occasionally referred pain from the thoracic cavity and mediastinum may potentially be responsible.

Fortunately, if a good history is available, a logical working diagnosis can usually be formulated with the benefit of basic physical examination and a small number of focused investigations.

As for any patient presenting acutely, the initial hurdle is determining his or her overall stability. In the context of acute abdominal pain look particularly for:

- *Signs of peritonism.*
- *Unstable clinical observations.*

If the patient is showing signs of instability, involve a senior at an early stage.

History: Employ the usual approach to a history, e.g. site, radiation, nature, intensity of pain. In addition, assess for the presence or absence of any other GI symptoms, such as vomiting, constipation, diarrhoea, melaena, and frank bleeding. Are there any urinary symptoms? If applicable, when was the last menstrual period? Is there any history of previous abdominal surgery?

Examination: Standard abdominal + rectal examination. Pay particular attention to tenderness and guarding.

Diagnoses not to miss

Keep the following in mind when assessing patients:

- **Abdominal aortic aneurysm (AAA):** Abdominal, loin, or back pain, signs of shock, pulsatile mass on examination, known to have AAA (on surveillance, etc.). Patients usually have risk factors for atheroma or suffer from related disease processes – IHD, etc.
- **Ectopic pregnancy:** Unilateral lower abdominal pain in the context of a positive beta human chorionic gonadotropin (βHCG) ± signs of shock.
- **Pancreatitis:** Epigastric or periumbilical abdominal pain, raised amylase or lipase, known gall stones, alcoholism. Presence of SIRS response.
- **Acute MI:** May occasionally present with epigastric pain – exercise a low threshold for 12-lead ECG in patients with risk factors for atheroma or known pre-existing ischaemic heart disease.
- **Ischaemic bowel:** Often a difficult diagnosis; usually acute onset of severe abdominal pain with raised serum lactate reflecting reduced gut perfusion. Aetiology may be thrombosis *in situ* (usually a consequence of atheroma) or embolic – atrial fibrillation (AF)/left ventricular (LV) thrombus, etc.

- **Appendicitis:** History of periumbilical pain that gradually localizes to the right iliac fossa as the inflamed appendix makes contact with the overlying parietal peritoneum. Patients may also have SIRS. Disease tends to affect the younger population, but not always.

Focused investigations

The investigations undertaken should always be tailored to the specifics of each patient, but the following are usually considered for the 'typical' patient with acute abdominal pain:

- Routine bloods: FBC, U&E, LFT, clotting.
- Serum amylase/lipase.
- Serum lactate.
- Urine dipstick + βHCG (perform in *all* females of childbearing age).
- Erect CXR (looking for free air under the diaphragm).
- AXR.

General management

- Keep nil by mouth (NBM) pending senior review.
- IV fluid (base prescription on volume status and U&E).
- Intravenous antibiotics (if indicated based on working diagnosis).
- Consider nasogastric (NG) tube (if persistently vomiting).
- Analgesia and anti-emetic as required.

Booking a patient for theatre

Following senior review it often falls to juniors to 'book' the patient for theatre. This involves speaking to the emergency theatre team and providing basic patient details, including the planned operation. The case is then added to the existing emergency list, which usually proceeds in chronological order.

Have the following to hand:

- Patient name/DOB/hospital ID.
- Planned operation.
- Fasting status.
- Allergy status.
- Any major issues – e.g. methicillin-resistant *Staphylococcus aureus* (MRSA) status, category C (HIV, hepatitis, etc.).

As part of the booking process, the surgical team must also discuss the case with the on-call anaesthetist. In addition to the above, the anaesthetist will be particularly interested in the following:

- **Body mass index (BMI):** Large patients are often problematic for anaesthetists.
- **Any significant PMH:** Particularly cardiac or respiratory pathology.

Acute causes of abdominal pain not to miss

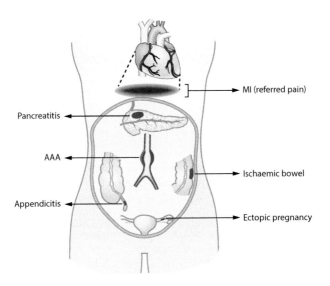

Key points

- Abdominal pain usually reflects pathology involving the intra-abdominal or pelvic organs.
- Referred pain is uncommon but always worth considering: acute MI can present with epigastric pain.
- Keep in mind the common, potentially life-threatening diagnoses for each patient you see.
- Booking a patient for the emergency theatre involves speaking to the theatre sister and on-call anaesthetist – have all relevant patient information to hand.

Sepsis is a complex syndrome with a very high mortality; patients who develop septic shock have a mere one in two chance of survival. As a result, there is a huge drive toward early recognition and prompt treatment of sepsis.

Essentially, sepsis is a severe generalized response to an infective process. This response was defined in 2001 as the systemic inflammatory response syndrome (SIRS), which has added diagnostic clarity to a process that was traditionally quite hard to define.

SIRS usually occurs in the context of infection (sepsis) but may also be triggered by non-infective causes: burns, trauma, etc. Patients are classed as having SIRS if they have two or more of the following:

- Body temperature of more than 38°C (100.4°F) or less than 36°C (96.8°F).
- Heart rate of more than 90 beats per minute.
- Respiratory rate of more than 20 breaths per minute or arterial carbon dioxide tension ($PaCO_2$) of less than 32mmHg.
- Abnormal white blood cell count (>12,000/µl or <4000/µl or >10% immature (band) forms).

With this in mind, the following definitions are well worth committing to memory:

Sepsis: SIRS in conjunction with a proven or assumed infection.

Severe sepsis: Sepsis with evidence of *inadequate organ perfusion* – altered mental state (CNS), oliguria (kidney), lactic acidosis (general marker of inadequate tissue perfusion).

Septic shock: Severe sepsis with hypotension refractory to fluid resuscitation.

> **The role of the F1:** Early recognition is key. Think SIRS whenever reviewing a patient with a new or ongoing infection. The initial management steps are outlined below.

The 'sepsis six'

These are the crucial first six management steps for the patient with sepsis as set out by the European Society of Critical Care Medicine. As an F1, these should form the basis of initial management, along with a focused history and examination to try and identify the source of infection.

1. **Give high-flow oxygen where appropriate.**
2. **Take blood cultures.**
3. **Give IV antibiotics.**
4. **Start fluid resuscitation.**
5. **Measure serum lactate.**
6. **Measure hourly urine output (usually requiring urinary catheter).**

Focused assessment

In addition to the above, assess thoroughly to try and establish the source of infection. Consider the following:

Respiratory: *Pneumonia or other respiratory infection.* SOB, increased work of breathing, cough, sputum production, haemoptysis, focal chest signs.

Urinary: *Lower UTI or pyelonephritis.* Dysuria, polyuria, haematuria, suprapubic pain, loin pain, long-term catheter?

Central nervous system: *Meningitis or encephalitis.* Headache, neck stiffness, photophobia, low GCS despite adequate BP, examine for Kernig's/Brudzinski's signs (although usually only positive with advanced infection).

Gastro-intestinal: *Intra-abdominal infection, perforated viscus/anastomotic leak.* Abdominal pain, diarrhoea, vomiting, recent/previous abdominal surgery, tenderness/guarding. New onset diarrhoea – any recent antibiotics; could this be a *Clostridium difficile* infection?

Cardiovascular system (CVS): *Endocarditis.* Evolving heart murmur, known valvular lesion, recent IV drug use, peripheral stigmata (splinter haemorrhages, Janeway lesions, etc.).

Lines: Examine all peripheral lines for signs of infection; usually manifest as erythema/swelling and soreness.

Skin: *Bed sores and superficial skin infections.* Examine top to toe.

Despite thorough clinical assessment, it is not always possible to immediately locate the focal source. In this situation a number of investigations are performed to try and establish the site of infection, a process referred to as a 'septic screen'. The exact investigations undertaken will vary somewhat depending on the specifics of the case, but the following would be typical:

- **CXR:** Performed in the vast majority.
- **Urine dip:** Quick and simple, should be performed on all patients with sepsis. Dip the urine for leukocytes and nitrites, if positive consider commencing treatment for UTI and send the sample for microscopy, culture and sensitivity.
- **Line cultures:** Check all lines for signs of infection. Cultures can be taken from arterial lines, central lines and peripherally inserted central catheters (PICC lines) if these are thought to be responsible. Consider re-siting any line thought to be the trigger for an infective process as a clinical priority.
- **Sputum cultures:** Send sputum cultures where possible, but this is obviously not feasible if the patient is not expectorating.
- **Swabs:** Swab any open wounds – bed sores, diabetic ulcers, etc.
- **Cardiac echocardiography:** Order where infective endocarditis is suspected; this is usually a senior decision.

Key points

- Sepsis is very common in clinical practice.
- Early recognition and management improve outcome.
- Consider the diagnosis of SIRS/sepsis for any patient with a presumed or known infection.
- The 'sepsis 6' are the crucial basic management steps to be undertaken for all patients with sepsis.
- Try to establish the focal source utilizing a combination of history, examination and a 'septic screen' where indicated.

One aspect of on-call medical work is responding to cardiac arrest calls across the hospital. You will be part of a cardiac arrest team which is usually directed by the senior doctor present. The majority of in-hospital cardiac arrests are either pulseless electrical activity (PEA) or asystole, and only a very small percentage survive to discharge.

The UK Resuscitation Council sets out specific guidelines for the management of cardiac arrest under the umbrella term *advanced life support*, the basic algorithm for which is displayed later in this chapter. It is well worth committing this to memory before starting out as an F1.

In essence, the majority of cardiac arrest management is very straightforward. There is no substitute for undertaking an official advanced life support (ALS) course, but the following tips will hopefully be of benefit when starting out on the wards.

Arriving at an arrest

The initial management steps should be as follows:

- Confirm cardiac arrest.
- Begin high-quality chest compressions (30:2 ratio).
- Ventilate the patient with a 'bag and mask' (usually 'Ambu®' breathing system). (If confident and trained, LMA or Igel can be used.)
- Attach the defibrillator; assess the rhythm and act accordingly.

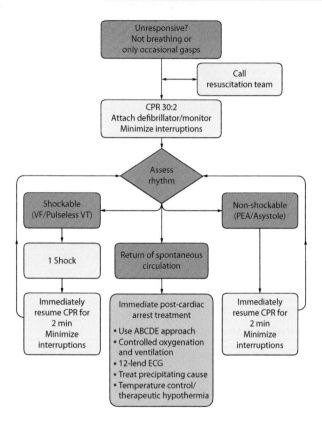

ALS Algorithm

Reproduced with permission from the Resuscitation Council, UK.

- Assign someone the task of timing each 2-minute cycle.
- Secure IV access – ideally 2, as big as possible.
- Start IV fluid – crystalloid (but not 5% dextrose!).
- Obtain an arterial blood gas and measure blood glucose.
- Measure core body temperature.

Things you want to know

In addition to the interventions above, it is important to establish certain key pieces of information from the nursing staff. Consider asking the following when it is possible to do so:

- Was the collapse witnessed or unwitnessed?
- If witnessed, what exactly happened?
- Any preceding symptoms? (Chest pain, SOB, palpitations, abdominal pain, etc.)
- Estimated 'downtime'. (How long has the patient been arrested? Very important prognostically.)
- Age of patient and past medical history.
- Why is the patient in hospital?
- Any recent notable events in care.
- Allergy status.
- Pre-morbid status: what was the patient's level of function prior to admission to hospital?

The new F1

As an F1 your role will usually involve chest compressions or establishing IV access. However, if you are the first to arrive at an arrest, there is no reason why an F1 doctor cannot adopt a leadership role if he or she has undertaken an ALS course.

Practical tips

- Ensure the bed is moved away from the wall and remove the bed head. This allows access to the airway.
- Ensure the bed is flat.
- Talk to the other team members. Communication is a key feature of successful cardiac arrest management.

Typical cardiac arrest scenario

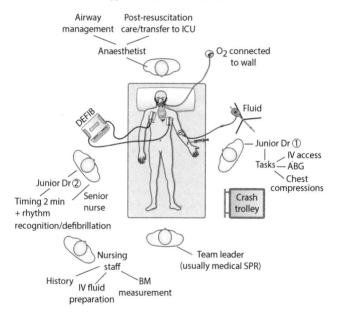

Key points

- On arrival at the bedside, confirm the diagnosis of cardiac arrest.
- Make sure the team has enough space to work – bedheads and tables may have to be removed from the bed space.
- Follow the ALS algorithm – try to commit this to memory before starting on-call work.
- Establish the sequence of events leading up to the arrest by speaking to nursing staff/witnesses.
- Communicate calmly and effectively with the rest of the cardiac arrest team.

As an F1, you will often be asked to assess patients who have fallen on the wards. The majority will be elderly patients who have sustained 'mechanical' falls with no major consequences, but don't get caught out! Examine each patient thoroughly. The assessment can be considered in three parts:

1. A, B, C, D, E assessment.
2. Establishing the cause for the fall if possible.
3. Identifying and treating any physical injury.

Establishing the cause

Establishing the cause for the fall may be easier said than done, particularly if the patient is elderly and unable to give an accurate account of what happened. The main aim, if possible, is to distinguish between a fall that is mechanical, i.e. a trip or momentary loss of balance, and a fall due to a medical cause, such as an arrhythmia or a stroke, for example.

- Take a history. Does the patient recall what happened? Did he or she trip? Lose balance? Or were there any symptoms prior to the fall – dizziness, chest pain, palpitations, SOB, headache, weakness, etc. Does he or she have pain anywhere?
- Did the nursing staff witness the fall?
- Take into account the patient's medical history, why he or she is in the hospital, and any recent events in his or her care.

- Examine the patient thoroughly: cardiovascular, respiratory, musculoskeletal, neurological, GI and document your findings.

Physical injuries not to miss

Head injury:

- General observation for abrasions, lacerations, soft tissue swelling.
- Check the drug card. Is the patient on warfarin or any other anticoagulants?
- Palpate the head and occiput.
- Assess the cranial nerves.
- Check ears and nose for signs of basal skull fracture. Look for Battle's sign and racoon sign.
- Assess GCS.
- All patients with a head injury should receive regular neurological observations (neuro OBS) for a set period – hospitals usually have a protocol for this.
- Consider a CT head for patients with a drop in their GCS, focal neurology, ongoing warfarin therapy, or clotting disorders.
- Close any lacerations with surgical glue or skin sutures.

Hip/pubic rami fracture:

- Fully assess the hips and pelvis in any elderly patient who has fallen: Can they straight leg raise?
- Exercise a very low threshold for hip + pelvic x-rays – elderly patients may not be able to localize their pain or present in a textbook fashion.

- If patients are complaining of pain, make sure you address their analgesia as well as diagnosing the cause.

Chest injury: pneumothorax/haemothorax

- Examine the chest for clinical signs of the above.
- If you suspect either diagnosis; give supplemental oxygen if hypoxaemia is present, request an urgent CXR and call for senior help.

Key points

- Falls remain common amongst the elderly population in hospital.
- Aim to identify both the cause and any physical injury sustained.
- Common injuries not to miss include: head injury, chest injury and fractures involving the hips and pelvis.
- Head injuries of any significance warrant regular neuro OBS – usually set out by local protocol.
- Exercise a low threshold for x-raying the hips of elderly patients following a fall.

Transfusion of blood products is a common practice in acute hospital trusts. As an F1, it will often fall to you to prescribe the products, and you are likely to be the first doctor consulted when a transfusion-related complication arises. Clinical features will vary depending on the exact nature of the reaction. Broadly speaking, keep a look out for *fever, urticaria, SOB,* or *CVS instability* that occurs specifically after the onset of transfusion.

Complications of transfusion may occur as a result of allergy, SIRS response, or may manifest as a respiratory complication. These are grouped into specific clinical entities, as follows.

Allergy

Allergic reactions tend to occur soon after starting the transfusion.

- *Mild allergic reactions* usually present with urticaria. Providing the patient is otherwise well, treat with chlorphenamine 10mg as a slow IV bolus, slow the rate of the transfusion and increase the frequency of clinical observations.
- *Anaphylaxis* to blood products is uncommon. In the event of this occurring: call for help, stop the transfusion immediately, and treat as for any anaphylactic reaction.

SIRS

SIRS-related reactions are classified as:

- **Febrile, non-haemolytic transfusion reactions:** This form of reaction occurs in 1–2% of transfusions and causes an isolated fever in an otherwise stable patient. If core body temperature rises up to 1.5°C above baseline, give paracetamol 1g, slow the rate of the transfusion, and increase the frequency of clinical observations. If the temperature exceeds 1.5°C, get senior help as a priority.
- **Acute haemolytic reactions and bacterial contamination reaction:** Both types tend to present in a similar fashion, with an acute, severe reaction characterized by cardiovascular instability or collapse, the onset of which is usually immediately after commencing the transfusion. Haemolytic reactions occur due to incompatible blood products being given to a patient. This is the result of an iatrogenic error at some point in the cross-matching/transfusion process. Bacterial contamination reactions are extremely rare and are the result of viable bacteria within the blood product itself.

If a severe reaction occurs, undertake the following:

- Stop the transfusion immediately and send to the laboratory for examination.
- A, B, C, D, E assessment and summon senior help/crash team.
- High-flow oxygen.
- IV access and fluid resuscitation.
- Blood cultures.

- IV antibiotics: Discuss with microbiology at the earliest opportunity; if advice isn't immediately available, follow local protocol for neutropenic sepsis. (Antibiotics are not theoretically needed for a haemolytic reaction, but in an acute setting it is usually impossible to distinguish between the two phenomena.)
- Critical care and haematology input.
- Don't forget: Address the initial indication for transfusion once the patient has stabilized.

Respiratory-related complications

Two forms of complications are recognized:

- **TRALI:** Transfusion-related acute lung injury. This is ARDS, secondary to blood transfusion.
- **TACO:** Transfusion-associated cardiovascular overload.

Patients in both groups will present with the typical features of acute respiratory compromise. TRALI has a typical onset time of 6 hours after commencement of the transfusion; TACO tends to develop more rapidly. However, in the initial stages it may be difficult to distinguish between the two.

Initial management is centred on the principles of any acute respiratory emergency:

- Sit upright.
- High-flow oxygen as indicated.
- ABG, bloods, CXR, etc.

In addition, patients suffering from TACO should receive IV loop diuretics (as for acute left ventricular failure).

Key points

- Transfusion reactions may manifest as an allergic reaction, SIRS response or respiratory complication.
- Allergic reactions usually present with urticaria but anaphylaxis may occasionally occur.
- SIRS-related reactions maybe subcategorized as: febrile non-haemolytic, acute haemolytic, and reactions secondary to bacterial contamination.
- Respiratory complications are defined as either TRALI (acute lung injury secondary to blood products) or TACO (volume overload resulting from transfusion).

Hyperkalaemia is a relatively common and potentially fatal electrolyte abnormality. Left untreated, it can adversely affect the myocardium causing dysrhythmias and ultimately cardiac arrest. As such, severe hyperkalaemia demands immediate management and close monitoring.

Causes

These may be subcategorized as follows:

- **Oliguric renal failure**.
- **Reduced aldosterone:** Angiotensin-converting enzyme inhibitor (ACEi), angiotensin receptor blockers (ARBs), spironolactone, amiloride.
- **Excess potassium:** Supplementation, rhabdomyolysis, tumour breakdown.
- **Transmembrane shift:** Acidosis, digoxin/suxamethonium.

Whilst the potential causes are numerous, in the context of general medical/surgical wards you are most likely to see hyperkalaemia as a result of renal failure, acidosis, and in the presence of drugs that affect the renin-angiotensin-aldosterone system.

When to treat

Treat hyperkalaemia if K$^+$ >6mmol/L or >5.3mmol/L *with* ECG changes. (ECG: Look for flattened or absent P-waves, wide QRS, tall-tented T-waves.)

Management

The treatment of hyperkalaemia is centred on:

- Protection of the myocardium.
- Moving potassium intracellularly.
- Treating the cause or removing precipitating factors where possible.
- Removal of potassium from the body.

Treatment

- **A, B, C, D, E.**
- **Perform 12-lead ECG.**
- **Protect the myocardium:** Give 10ml of 10% calcium gluconate as an IV bolus over 2 minutes. If ECG changes persist, the dose may be repeated every 15 minutes up to a total of 50ml. Connect patient to heart monitor before giving the bolus; this allows visual confirmation that the ECG has normalized.
- **Move potassium intracellularly:** Two main methods are used: Give salbutamol via nebulizer. The onset of action is approximately 15 minutes with a duration of 2 hours. This is simple and quick to set up in a hurry. Commence an infusion of insulin and dextrose; the exact dose of insulin and concentration and volume of dextrose is

usually dictated by local protocol, but the following would be fairly standard: 10 units of actrapid in 50ml of 50% dextrose given as an IVI over 15 minutes. The onset is 15 minutes with a duration of action between 4 and 6 hours.

- **Treat the cause or remove precipitating factors:** Take a history, examine the patient, assess bloods and review the drug Kardex to try and establish the cause. Omit ACE inhibitors, ARBs, spironolactone, amiloride, and digoxin for 24 hours if your senior is in agreement. Treat acute kidney injury with IV fluid and insert a urinary catheter.
- **Remove potassium from the body:** Prescribe Calcium Resonium® 15g orally four times a day or alternatively provide as an enema. Resins exchange ions in the GI tract.
- **General management:** All patients should have a full set of bloods sent and labelled as urgent. Involve a senior doctor at an early stage, particularly in the presence of marked ECG changes or if the patient has additional complexities, such as ongoing digoxin therapy.

General considerations

In addition to the steps outlined in the treatment section, keep the following in mind when treating patients with hyperkalaemia:

- Is the result expected or seemingly random? If there is any doubt about the result, check by obtaining an ABG or venous gas in addition to a repeat U&E. This will give you an answer quickly.

- Beware patients taking digoxin: Giving calcium gluconate may precipitate myocardial digoxin toxicity. If necessary, dilute in 100ml 0.9% saline and give as an infusion over 20 minutes. Seek senior advice before commencing.
- Hyperkalaemia with co-existing hypoxia carries a greater risk of conduction abnormalities.
- The ECG may demonstrate no changes despite significant hyperkalaemia; a 'normal' ECG does not negate the need for treatment.
- The use of venous bicarbonate has long been a traditional treatment for hyperkalaemia. However, up-to-date guidance does not recommend its routine use in this context.

Causes of hyperkalaemia

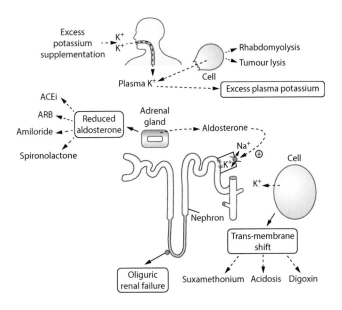

Key points

- Hyperkalaemia may cause cardiac arrest.
- The most common causes include oliguric renal failure, acidosis and drugs that act on the renin–angiotensin aldosterone system.
- Treat when K^+ > 6mmol/L or > 5.3mmol/L with ECG changes.
- Basic treatment should include: protecting the myocardium with calcium gluconate, moving K^+ intra-cellularly with insulin and salbutamol, and removing K^+ from the body with Calcium Resonium.
- Aim to treat or reverse the underlying cause where possible.

Strokes, or cerebrovascular accidents (CVAs), represent a significant cause of morbidity and mortality with an average incidence of 1/100 in those aged greater than 75. Patients with an established CVA are usually cared for on designated stroke units, which provide specialist medical, nursing, and therapy input.

In the acute setting, the main clinical challenges are:

- Determining whether the CVA is the result of ischaemic infarction or intra-cerebral (IC) haemorrhage.
- If *ischaemic*, is the patient suitable for thrombolysis?
- If *haemorrhagic*, would the patient benefit from neurosurgical intervention?

Ischaemic CVA

These account for 80% of all strokes and are the result of either a thrombosis superimposed upon an atherosclerotic plaque within a cerebral artery (most common) or an embolic event. Vasculitis, thrombocytosis or fibromuscular dysplasia may occasionally be responsible. Common embolic sources include those of cardiac origin: arrhythmias predisposing to thrombus formation, left ventricular (LV) thrombus, endocarditis and also atherothrombotic lesions embolizing from the carotid arteries.

Ischaemic CVAs are subcategorized based on the artery they involve, e.g. middle cerebral artery (MCA) infarct (see diagram). Occlusion of each vessel should theoretically give rise to a particular neurological deficit depending on the function of the brain parenchyma supplied by the vessel. However, the clinical signs are often clouded by collateral supply from other vessels, atypical anatomy etc.

The onset of symptoms can vary significantly and doesn't always follow a predictable pattern. In theory, a true embolic stroke will produce a very acute onset of symptoms with maximal neurological deficit seen immediately, whereas an infarct caused by thrombosis *in situ* tends to develop over minutes to hours.

Haemorrhagic CVA

These represent the remaining 20% of acute strokes. Presentation is usually with acute onset of neurological signs accompanied or preceded by severe headache (although not in every case). Examination findings usually reveal focal neurology ± signs of rising intracranial pressure (ICP). Common causes include hypertension, anticoagulation states (warfarin, recent thrombolysis), aneurysm/ arteriovenous malformation (AVM) rupture, and trauma. Subarachnoid haemorrhage (SAH) is a specific form of haemorrhagic CVA caused by bleeding into the subarachnoid space as a result of either berry aneurysm rupture (85%) or AVM (15%). They are associated with both connective tissue and polycystic disease. SAHs generally affect a younger population and are often amenable to surgical or radiological intervention.

Management

- A, B, C, D, E.
- IV access.
- Keep NBM pending swallow assessment.
- Maintenance fluid as an intravenous infusion.
- Bloods: FBC, U&E, LFT, clotting, erythrocyte sedimentation rate (ESR), vasculitic screen.
- ECG + CXR.
- Organize bed on stroke unit.
- CT head (or appropriate brain imaging – MRI in some centres).
  - If haemorrhage is demonstrated on imaging, a senior doctor will discuss with the neurosurgical team to determine whether any form of intervention is possible. Any clotting derangement should be corrected at this time.
  - If no haemorrhage is identified on the initial scan, a working diagnosis of ischaemic stroke can be made. Treatment should commence with either thrombolysis (if indicated) or a loading dose of aspirin 300mg given PR.
- Ideally all patients presenting with an acute stroke should be managed on a designated stroke unit.

When to image

In the context of acute stroke, imaging should be obtained as soon as possible. The speed with which a head CT or brain MRI can be obtained may vary between trusts but ideally should be undertaken as a clinical priority. At the very least, all patients should receive a scan within 24 hours of admission to the hospital.

Thrombolysis for ischaemic stroke

Thrombolysis with alteplase is considered for patients with acute ischaemic stroke, with no evidence of haemorrhage, who present within a 4.5-hour window from symptom onset. This time frame was increased from 3 to 4.5 hours in March 2012. *As an F1, an important part of your role will be quickly highlighting to seniors any patient who falls into this bracket.*

Contraindications: As with any form of thrombolytic therapy, the list of contraindications to stroke thrombolysis is considerable. Unless you work on a stroke unit, this information shouldn't be expected of new F1s.

**A little anatomy — patterns of focal
neurology seen with ischaemic strokes**

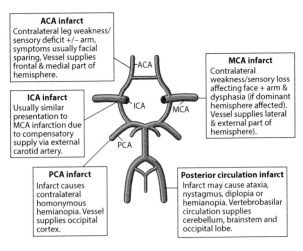

ACA infarct
Contralateral leg weakness/
sensory deficit +/– arm,
symptoms usually facial
sparing, Vessel supplies
frontal & medial part of
hemisphere.

MCA infarct
Contralateral
weakness/sensory loss
affecting face + arm &
dysphasia (if dominant
hemisphere affected).
Vessel supplies lateral
& external part of
hemisphere).

ICA infarct
Usually similar
presentation to
MCA infarction due
to compensatory
supply via external
carotid artery.

PCA infarct
Infarct causes
contralateral
homonymous
hemianopia. Vessel
supplies occipital
cortex.

Posterior circulation infarct
Infarct may cause ataxia,
nystagmus, diplopia or
hemianopia. Vertebrobasilar
circulation supplies
cerebellum, brainstem and
occipital lobe.

ACA – anterior cerebral artery; ICA – internal carotid artery;
MCA – middle cerebral artery; PCA – posterior cerebral artery.

Stroke aetiology

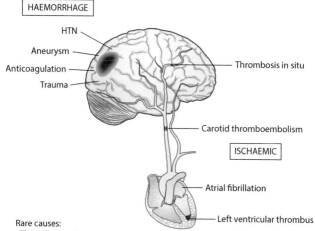

HAEMORRHAGE

HTN

Aneurysm

Anticoagulation

Trauma

Thrombosis in situ

Carotid thromboembolism

ISCHAEMIC

Atrial fibrillation

Left ventricular thrombus

Rare causes:
- Thrombocytosis
- Vasculitis
- Fibromuscular dysplasia
- Endocarditis

Key points

- Strokes are categorized as ischaemic or haemorrhagic depending upon the underlying pathology.
- Appropriate brain imaging (usually head CT) should be undertaken at the earliest opportunity.
- Haemorrhagic strokes are usually discussed with the neurosurgical team to decide whether surgery or interventional radiology is appropriate.
- Patients who suffer an ischaemic stroke are offered thrombolysis if they present within 4.5 hours of symptom onset in the absence of any contra-indications. The remainder are treated with aspirin.

Low urine output 'oliguria' is defined clinically as an output less than or equal to **0.5ml/kg/hour**.

Great clinical emphasis is placed upon maintaining a 'normal' urine output, and for good reason: the presence of oliguria implies a degree of impairment to normal renal function, the severity of which increases with the duration of the oliguric episode.

Acute kidney injury (AKI) can be classified both by cause and by severity.

Cause

The potential causes are traditionally subcategorized into three groups, although quite often the aetiology is mixed:

- **Pre-renal:** Any cause resulting in reduced renal perfusion.
- **Intra-renal:** Any intrinsic kidney insult.
- **Post-renal:** Any obstruction distal to the kidney.

Pre-renal: These causes are the most common in the general hospital population. Reduced perfusion may result from any form of cardiovascular instability, including low cardiac output states (LVF, MI, PE), hypovolaemia (blood loss, dehydration, third space loss), and conditions such as sepsis where vasodilation and third space loss occur in combination.

Intra-renal: This group includes a wide mix of causes, most of which are quite rare and seen most frequently by renal teams. On general wards, intrinsic causes are most often a result of drug nephrotoxicity. In particular, check the drug Kardex for aminoglycosides, NSAIDs, ACE inhibitors, and metformin. Involve a senior when deciding whether or not to omit potentially nephrotoxic drugs.

Post-renal: These causes encompass any form of mechanical obstruction distal to the kidney. Common examples include obstruction of an existing urinary catheter, prostatic disease, and ureteric calculi.

Severity

Severity is commonly described by use of the RIFLE classification system. This scoring system places patients into one of five groups based on the severity of oliguria or degree of rise in plasma creatinine level above normal levels for the patient:

R = Risk: Output less than or equal to 0.5ml/kg/hour for 6 hours or serum creatinine 1.5 times baseline.

I = Injury: Output less than or equal to 0.5ml/kg/hour for 12 hours or serum creatinine two times baseline.

F = Failure: Output less than or equal to 0.3ml/kg/hour for 24 hours or serum creatinine three times baseline.

L = Loss: Complete loss of function greater than 4 weeks.

E = End stage: Requiring dialysis.

An approach to management

The exact management will depend very much on the presumed aetiology of the oliguria and whether or not steps can be taken to reverse the underlying pathology. In all patients, ask yourself the following:

Assessment:

- Does the patient appear volume depleted? (HR, BP, turgor, mucous membranes, postural BP drop, thirst)
- Is he or she drinking?
- Any evidence of sepsis?
- Any pre-existing renal disease?
- Any known obstructive disorders? (BPH, ureteric calculi, etc.)
- Any symptoms/signs suggesting CCF, MI, or PE?
- Is the patient receiving drugs with potential for nephrotoxicity?

Treatment:

- Treat any obvious cause, e.g. infection.
- Treat hyperkalaemia if present.
- Bloods: FBC, U&E + blood cultures if sepsis suspected.
- Insert a urinary catheter if one is not already present and request close and accurate monitoring of the urine output.
- Give a fluid challenge: 500ml IV crystalloid initially and assess response (response may not be immediate).
- Check the drug Kardex for the presence of nephrotoxic drugs.

- Request a renal ultrasound scan (USS) to look for an obstructive cause if the aetiology is uncertain. This is usually done in daylight hours.
- Involve a senior and reassess the patient following the above interventions.
- Obtain an arterial blood gas to assess acid–base balance.

Causes of acute kidney injury

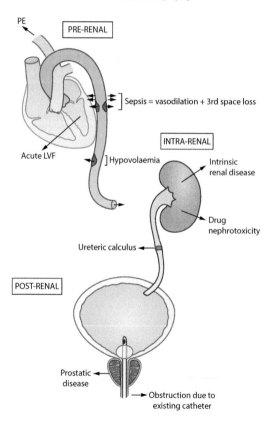

PE

PRE-RENAL

Sepsis = vasodilation + 3rd space loss

INTRA-RENAL

Acute LVF

Hypovolaemia

Intrinsic renal disease

Drug nephrotoxicity

Ureteric calculus

POST-RENAL

Prostatic disease

Obstruction due to existing catheter

Key points

- Oliguria is defined as a urine output less than or equal to 0.5ml/kg/hr.
- Both the cause and severity are important to consider for patients with AKI.
- Causes are traditionally considered as pre-renal, intra-renal or post-renal, with pre-renal causes being the most common.
- Severity can be assessed using the RIFLE criteria.

Section C

Situations and communication

Microbiology is a medical specialty dealing with complex infections. Your main encounters as an F1 will be discussing patients with the on-call microbiologist to determine the most appropriate antibiotic therapy. Certain antibiotics also require a 'code' to be provided by microbiology before they can be prescribed. This comprises a series of numbers and letters which must be documented on the drug card. Before ringing micro, make sure you know the following:

- Basic patient details.
- Site of infection (pneumonia, UTI, etc.).
- Antibiotic therapy so far.
- Any allergies to antibiotics (make sure you know the type of reaction if possible).
- Recent antibiotic courses.
- Recent blood results – particularly white cell count (WCC) and inflammatory markers.
- Any recent culture results.
- Body temperature and observations (OBS).

It is essential to document the conversation in the clinical notes. If a code has been given, make sure you also write this in the clinical notes; drug cards have a habit of getting lost.

An important part of on call (and ward work in general) is being able to present patients to senior colleagues, either for advice or to request a review of the patient. This can seem daunting when starting out as an F1. There is no right or wrong way to go about this, but having a framework that you are comfortable with is useful.

Things to consider include:

- Age, gender, and location of patient.
- Why the patient was admitted to the hospital.
- Outline of past medical history (PMHx).
- Why you were called to review the patient.
- Any notable events in their treatment/management.
- Details of your assessment and treatment so far.
- Your request for the senior clinician.

It's important to be specific when requesting help or advice. If you need your senior to review the patient rather than discuss over the phone, make that clear early on.

For example: 'I wonder if you could review a 60-year-old lady with chest pain on ward A2....'

If you are discussing over the phone, make sure you have the patient's notes, drug card, OBS chart and recent investigation results next to you when making the call.

The majority of chest x-rays (CXRs) are taken in the hospital's main radiology department, both during the day and also out of hours. On occasions, patients may be too unstable to leave a ward or clinical area, and in this situation the radiographer will come directly to the ward and take the CXR using a portable machine.

There are no hard-and-fast rules, but consider requesting a portable CXR in the following circumstances:

- Any peri-arrest patient.
- Patients requiring immediate treatment (boluses of furosemide or nebulizers, for example).
- Any patient with signs of acute respiratory distress.
- Patients with cardiovascular instability.

Ultimately, the decision comes down to clinical judgement on a case-by-case basis. If you aren't sure, check with a senior.

When requesting a portable CXR:

- Ensure you ring the on-call radiographer to confirm the request.
- Give a brief summary of why the patient is unable to travel to the x-ray department.
- Most departments require a paper request to be completed.

- Give the radiographer a hand positioning the patient – this is appreciated!

When patients pass away on the wards a trained clinician needs to examine the patient to confirm that he or she has died. In some hospitals senior nursing staff are trained to do this, but often the task falls to the F1 doctor.

Essentially, this involves a basic clinical examination to confirm that the patient has died.

The following would be a standard approach:

- Listen for heart sounds for 1 minute.
- Check for absence of a central pulse for 1 minute.
- Listen for breath sounds for 1 minute.
- Assess for any response to a painful stimulus (usually squeezing a finger).
- Check that the pupils are fixed and dilated using a pen torch.

In reality, it is usually obvious from general inspection that the patient has died, but a formal examination is expected in each case.

Document your examination in the clinical notes, making sure you note the time of your assessment – legally this is the time that the patient died.

When you start out, certifying deceased patients can be an unsettling experience, particularly when working out of hours on unfamiliar wards. As with anything else, you get used to it. Nursing staff are generally very supportive and will often come with you when you assess the patient.

Following acute admission to hospital, all patients will be reviewed by a consultant on a post-take ward round (PTWR). The format of this will vary somewhat between hospitals, but will usually take place once in every 24-hour period, usually starting first thing in the morning.

When covering medicine, the consultant may be a specialist working solely on the acute admissions unit (consultant in acute medicine), or the responsibility may be shared amongst all the medical consultants on a shared basis. Surgical consultants will generally share the post-take responsibility.

As with any ward round, F1 doctors play a key role. Whilst the management decisions and treatment plans are generally the responsibility of senior doctors, the general organisation and smooth running of the PTWR is usually considered to be the F1's responsibility. Consider the following:

- **Know your patients:** It's impossible to know everything, but try to have a working knowledge of each patient, particularly if you clerked the patient! E.g. working diagnosis, treatment, note-worthy abnormal investigations, etc.
- **Know where your patients are:** Create a list of all the patients to be seen along with their ward and bed space. Plan the ward round so that patients are seen in a logical order wherever possible.

- **Keep a job list:** Note jobs to be done at the bedside (e.g. order ECG, add thyroid-stimulating hormone (TSH) to bloods) and have a system for crossing jobs off after completion.
- **Communicate with nursing staff:** In most cases, the nurse looking after the patient will be present, but not always. Make sure the consultant plan is communicated to the nursing staff, even if this means returning to speak to the nurses after the ward round has finished.
- **Check the observation chart and drug Kardex:** The consultant will want to review both of these for each patient. Make sure you have these to hand when reviewing the patient.
- **Get the patients' notes out:** Be ready to document what has been said on the ward round and the plan for that day.

Overall, the key is to be organized and have a system that works for you. Consultants usually expect a brisk, efficient ward round with junior doctors having a good working knowledge of the patients.

PTWR Crib Sheet . . .

Bay 3: (MAU 1)

	BED 1	BED 4	

Mr. Smith: Δ NSTEMI

- Repeat ECG ☐
- Order ECHO ☑

Mr. Singh: Δ Sepsis ? source

- Repeat lactate ☐
- D/w critical care ☑

BED 2 / BED 5

Mr. Jones: Δ Pneumonia

- Discuss with micro ☐
- Chase cultures ☑
- Prescribe O$_2$ ▦

Mr. Patel: Δ Acute CVA

- Order Dopplers ☐
- Chase bloods ☑

BED 3 / BED 6

Mr. Murphy: Δ COPD exac

- Chase CxR ☐
- Switch NEBS to PRN ☑

Mr. Kahn: Δ Acute GI bleed

- Consent for OGD ☐
- Order group & save ☑

Triangle = working diagnosis.

Blood bank

The blood bank is a vital department found in all
acute hospital trusts and forms part of the haematology
directorate. In essence, the department is a laboratory
staffed by technicians and scientists with input from clinical
haematologists as required. The main responsibilities of
blood bank are twofold:

- To receive blood sample requests from across the hospital,
  e.g. group and screen.
- To store and dispense blood products as needed.

As a junior doctor, your involvement may vary from
drawing blood to enable cross-matching, to prescribing and
overseeing a transfusion. Either way, you will find yourself
playing a key role.

Blood bank receives three main requests from medical
staff:

Group and save: This involves analysing the blood sample
to determine the patient's ABO group and screening the
sample for common antibodies. No blood product is set aside
for the patient at this stage, but a valid group and save will

reduce the time required for a formal cross-match to take place should this become necessary. As such, this request is made when the patient is stable but there is a chance blood products may be required in the near future. A typical example would be a patient admitted for elective surgery.

Cross-match: This involves the same process as outlined for group and save, with the inclusion of an additional step whereby donor and patient samples are mixed to look for possible reactions. A cross-match is a direct request for blood, and the number of units required must be stated at the time of the request. Blood is usually cross-matched prior to surgery where significant blood loss is expected, e.g. abdominal aortic aneurysm repair.

Electronic issue: This is essentially an extension of the group and save request. If two group and save samples are sent to the lab, then blood can be dispensed without performing a formal cross-match. Samples must be taken at least 15 minutes apart, ideally by different clinicians.

Blood products

The most common blood products you are likely to encounter are:

- Red cells (by far the most common).
- Fresh frozen plasma (FFP).
- Platelets.
- Cryoprecipitate.

Red cells: Red cells are stored and dispensed in plastic pouches holding a volume somewhere between 200 and 300ml. Red cells must be used within 6 hours at room temperature and are given as an infusion using specialized wide-bore giving sets. The threshold for transfusion is usually 8g/dl for the general patient population, or 10g/dl for patients with ischaemic heart disease, although the exact transfusion threshold may vary slightly between trusts. When considering the number of red cells to request, remember: one 'unit' of red cells will usually raise the haemoglobin (HB) by 1g/dl.

Platelets: Platelets are suspended in plasma in a volume similar to red cells. They are stored in the lab for a period of 2 days under continuous agitation to maintain their function. One bag of platelets will increase the count by around 10, and generally only one bag will be required at a given time. The decision to transfuse platelets is usually based upon the dual considerations of platelet count and the clinical context. For example, consider platelet transfusion if:

- Platelet count is *less than or equal to 10* in an otherwise stable patient.
- Platelet count is *less than or equal to 50* in the presence of active bleeding, coagulopathy, critical illness, or surgery.

Fresh frozen plasma: FFP is presented in 200ml bags and consists of clotting factors, albumin, and antibodies. FFP must be used immediately following delivery to the clinical area and is given at a dose of 15ml/kg (usually equates to three or four bags. Common situations in which FFP may be required include:

- Significant active bleeding requiring high numbers of red cell units (the exact threshold usually comes down to clinical judgement).
- Reversal of severe warfarin overdose.
- Disseminated intravascular coagulation.

Cryoprecipitate: The primary use of cryoprecipitate is to treat low fibrinogen levels. Whilst several different causes may potentially be responsible, hypofibrinogenaemia is seen most commonly in the context of massive blood transfusion and disseminated intravascular coagulation. The usual treatment threshold is a plasma level less than 0.8g/dl.

> **Remember:** When requesting a group and save or cross-match, forms must be handwritten in full; otherwise the sample will be rejected.

Massive transfusion protocol

Most hospitals now operate massive transfusion protocols (or similar). This is usually activated by dialling 2222 as for any other hospital emergency. The protocol is essentially a system of communication that expedites the delivery of urgent blood products to a patient with massive haemorrhage. In addition, upon activation, the haematologist on call is usually notified and is then available to advise and support the clinical team as required.

The specifics of each protocol will vary between trusts – it is well worth checking the system in place for your hospital.

Receiving a needlestick injury is no fun at all, but will happen to most of us at some point. It is important to remember that the risk of transmission of any blood-borne virus is exceptionally small, and in the vast majority of cases, a needlestick results in no serious consequences. The importance of wearing gloves should not be underestimated. For one, it is best practice and has been shown to reduce the risk of transmission, and two, it is nearly always, if not always, hospital policy.

If you to sustain a needlestick injury, take the following steps:

- Dispose of the sharp safely.
- Wash the affected hand/finger in warm water and encourage bleeding (continue for at least 10 minutes).
- Make sure you cover or dress the wound.

Most hospitals have set guidelines for what to do next, and they can usually be found on the hospital intranet. Essentially, a blood sample must be taken from yourself and the patient – both are sent to the lab and screened. In normal working hours the occupational health department is usually available to perform venepuncture on clinical staff; if the incident occurs out of hours, staff would usually attend the ED. A trained colleague should take the sample from the source patient.

It is also important to inform the patient about the incident, partly to make him or her aware of the event, but also with a view to gaining consent for his or her blood sample. Most hospitals advise clinicians to try and identify patients who are 'high risk' for blood-borne viruses – typically this would include intravenous drug users, patients known to be category 3, and those who have undergone a recent blood transfusion.

Section D

Prescribing

One of the major transitions from medical student to doctor is the ability to prescribe medication. Drug prescriptions form a central component of a junior doctor's daily workload and come with a significant level of responsibility.

The following tips apply to any medication you prescribe. Whilst most of this is hammered home toward the end of our training, these points may act as a useful reminder:

- Write legibly, in capitals (ideally), and with black ink only.
- Know the mode of action of every drug you prescribe.
- Be sure of the dose – look up in the British National Formulary (BNF) if there is any uncertainty.
- Sign each prescription with your signature/name and bleep or contact number.
- Check the patient's allergy status before prescribing any drug.
- Avoid the use of trade names (enoxaparin rather than Clexane® for example).
- Check the drug card for possible interactions before prescribing.
- Include a 'review date' whenever prescribing antibiotics.

In the hospital setting, medications and intravenous fluids are prescribed on a 'drug card' or 'treatment Kardex,' which acts as a record of both the prescription and the fact that the medication has been administered by a nurse.

Drug cards consist of different sections:

Front page: This contains basic patient information including name, DOB, unit number, etc. There is also a large box where any allergies may be documented. The final section (usually toward the bottom) is used for 'once only medications.' This is most often used in acute situations where medications need to be provided without delay, but usually not on a regular basis.

Inside pages 1 and 2 – regular medications: Any drug to be given to the patient on a regular basis (whether commenced in or out of hospital) is prescribed in this section. For each drug, there are spaces for significant details, including dose, frequency, minimum interval between doses, and the 'start date' (date of first administration) for the drug. Start dates are straightforward if you are commencing a medicine in the hospital – if you are prescribing regular medicines that were started by the patient's GP, it is usually acceptable to write 'OA' (on admission), which indicates that the patient was already taking the medication on admission to the hospital.

Page 4 – PRN medication: This section is used for any medication you think the patient is likely to require during his or her admission, but not frequently enough to be prescribed in the regular section of the Kardex. Examples might include analgesics, anti-emetics, laxatives, a GTN spray for a patient with occasional angina, or a salbutamol inhaler for an asthmatic admitted to the hospital for something other than an asthma exacerbation. Clearly, what you decide to prescribe in this section will vary depending on the individual patient, and the nature of his or her admission.

Pain relief is a crucial element of patient care and should be addressed for every patient you see.

For the purposes of prescribing analgesics, make sure you know the following about the pain you are treating:

- Intensity/severity: Knowledge of pain intensity will guide you when deciding upon the type, dose, and route for the analgesic. For example, a patient in 'agony' with acute abdominal pain will clearly require very different analgesics than a patient suffering from a sore throat.
- Likely origin: This may guide you when deciding upon a particular type of analgesic. For example, nonsteroidal anti-inflammatory drugs (NSAIDs) are particularly effective when treating pain of musculoskeletal origin, whilst opiates/opioids are more beneficial in the context of visceral pain.
- Any patient specific factors:
  - History of gastritis or chronic kidney disease (CKD)/ acute kidney injury (AKI)? (NSAIDs often avoided.)
  - Patient weight? (Allows dose calculation for IV opiates.)
  - Does the patient have an epidural? (Can this be topped up?)
  - Does the patient have a patient controlled analgesic device (PCA)? (Can a bolus be delivered?)

Analgesics are numerous and varied. They come in many different formulations, combinations, and with different modes of action. Whilst a comprehensive discussion is beyond the scope of this book, the following illustrates the more common analgesics you are likely to encounter in hospital.

Commonly used analgesics

Paracetamol: 1g, QDS 4°, PO/IV

Widely used agent both in hospital and in the community. It possesses analgesic and antipyretic properties via inhibition of a subtype of the cyclo-oxygenase enzyme. Any patient with pain should ideally receive regular paracetamol as a baseline. It may be administered orally, intravenously, and occasionally as a suppository. Paracetamol has a low side effect profile when given at the recommended dose, but is particularly toxic in an overdose situation. *Note:* For IV paracetamol the dose reduces to 500mg if the patient weighs less than 40kg (beware young and old women in particular)!

Codeine Phosphate: 15–60mg, QDS 4°, PO

Weak opioid analgesic often used in combination with paracetamol, either as separate tablets taken together or as a combined preparation, e.g. co-codamol®.
Low doses are most often used in the elderly population. Also consider the addition of a regular laxative whilst the patient is taking codeine phosphate.
Co-codamol is available only as an oral preparation and comes in three strengths:

- Co-codamol 8/500 (1g paracetamol + 16mg codeine).
- Co-codamol 15/500 (1g paracetamol + 30mg codeine).
- Co-codamol 30/500 (1g paracetamol + 60mg codeine).

(All are prescribed as two tablets to be taken every 4 to 6 hours – maximum QDS.)

Tramadol: 50–100mg, QDS 4°, PO/IV

Provides analgesia due to opioid properties and action at seratonergic pathways. Considered a step up from codeine in terms of analgesic potency. May be delivered orally or via IV injection.

Ibuprofen: 400mg, TDS 6°, PO (occasionally topical)

Commonly used NSAID. Particularly effective when treating musculoskeletal pain, but also used in combination with paracetamol/codeine (or tramadol) when treating pain of visceral origin. Topical NSAIDs are now first-line agents in the treatment of hand and knee osteoarthritis. As with all NSAIDs, beware patients with active gastritis, haematemesis, or acute/chronic kidney injury. To minimize the risk posed by NSAIDS, they should be taken with or after food (this can be written with your prescription).

Buscopan: 20mg, QDS 4°, PO – usually

Buscopan (hyoscine butylbromide) is sometimes used as an adjunct for patients with 'colicky' pain thought to be secondary to smooth muscle spasm. Situations where buscopan may be particularly beneficial include ureteric colic and irritable bowel syndrome.

Morphine

- **Intravenous:** 0.1–0.2mg/kg (usually up to around 10mg).
- **Subcutaneous:** 10mg (can be given as often as 1 or 2 hourly).
- **Oral 'oramorph':** 5–10ml (10mg in 5ml, given 1 or 2 hourly).

Morphine is a potent opiate widely used in hospital practice – it is considered the benchmark against which all other opiates/opioids are compared. Morphine may be administered via a number of different routes, although intravenous, subcutaneous, and oral are the most common. IV morphine is used for patients in severe pain and is usually given by a doctor (unless you are working in the emergency department, where many of the nurses are able to do this). Subcutaneous and oral administration is more commonly used on general wards – the exact preparations and guidance for prescriptions are likely to vary slightly between hospitals. Patients receiving regular morphine in a palliative care setting may sometimes require a 'breakthrough' dose to alleviate their symptoms. This dose should be calculated as ⅙th of the patient's total daily dose of morphine.

As with any opiate, morphine has a number of potential side effects, including:

- **Nausea and vomiting** – always prescribe an anti-emetic with morphine.
- **Respiratory depression** – more common after an IV dose.
- **Pruritis** – itching is quite common. Consider prescribing an antihistamine on the PRN side of the drug card.

A note about neuropathic pain

Sometimes pain is thought to be due to dysfunction of the nervous system rather than secondary to nociceptive stimulation. Patients suffering from neuropathic pain are often under the care of a pain specialist. Whilst you won't be expected to initiate a prescription, you may see the likes of gabapentin, pregabalin, and amitriptyline used to treat this patient group.

Epidurals and PCAs

Epidurals

These are sited by anaesthetists in theatre, usually for patients undergoing major abdominal surgery, but are increasingly being used for the management of fractured ribs. An epidural is essentially a very thin plastic catheter which is positioned within the epidural space. The catheter is connected to a pump via a bacterial filter, which is then used to deliver a solution of local anaesthetic (often in combination with fentanyl or diamorphine) to the patient at a set rate in ml/hour. Some newer pumps incorporate a button which is controlled by the patient and allows further boluses of local anaesthetic to be delivered as required. If a patient with an epidural has poor pain control, it is worth contacting either the on-call anaesthetist or acute pain team for an assessment.

PCA

Patient controlled analgesic devices (PCAs) are essentially a morphine syringe driver which is under the control of the patient via a button. Activating the button delivers a bolus of drug followed by a lockout period (usually 5 minutes) to avoid accidental overdose. Patients with a PCA require an IV fluid prescription to keep the line patent.

Nausea and vomiting is something all of us can relate to, and to many members of the public, 'being sick' is almost the definition of illness. We are fortunate as hospital doctors in that we have many agents at our immediate disposal that can play an important role in the management of a patient who is vomiting.

However, anti-emetics are only part of the solution. When a patient is vomiting, ask yourself the following:

- **Why is the patient vomiting?** Probably the most important to establish – treat the cause where possible. For example, a patient with a small bowel obstruction will respond better to a nasogastric (NG) tube than an anti-emetic. Strictly speaking, an anti-emetic should only be prescribed once a working diagnosis has been made.
- **Is an anti-emetic indicated?** Anti-emetics will be beneficial in the majority of situations you will encounter; however, in the context of acute poisoning, use of anti-emetics may actually be detrimental.
- **Which anti-emetic is most appropriate?** Ideally, once the cause of the vomiting is known, the most logical anti-emetic is chosen, taking into account the cause for the vomiting (see below).

Common anti-emetics

As for analgesics, anti-emetics are a diverse group of
agents with a variety of modes of action. The following are
commonly used in hospital practice.

Antihistamines

The most obvious example is cyclizine. Cinnarizine and
promethazine may occasionally be used. Antihistamines
act on receptors both in the GI tract and on the vestibular
nucleus. As such, they are particularly effective in the
treatment of emesis resulting from gastrointestinal pathology
or problems with the inner ear/vestibular apparatus.
Potential side effects of cyclizine include sedation and
tachycardia (due to an anticholinergic effect.)

  Cyclizine, 50mg, TDS 6°, IV/IM/PO

Dopamine antagonists

This group includes a number of drugs, including the
phenothiazines (chlorpromazine, prochlorperazine),
metoclopramide and domperidone. All work by antagonist
activity at the D2 receptor (located in the GI tract) and the
chemoreceptor trigger zone (CTZ) and are thus effective
for vomiting due to a precipitant in the bloodstream (drugs,
acidosis, uraemia) and pathology involving the GI tract.
The main risk with dopamine antagonists is the phenomenon
of acute dystonia, more common with extremes of age
and female gender. For this reason, dopamine antagonists
are usually avoided in young females. In the event of an
acute dystonic reaction, the reversal agent is procyclidine.

Domperidone does not cross the blood brain barrier and is therefore less likely to precipitate a dystonic crisis.

Metoclopramide 10mg, TDS 6°, IV/IM/PO*

Domperidone 10–20mg, QDS 4°, PO*

Prochlorperazine 12.5mg, one-off IM injection (or PO)

5HT₃ antagonists

These drugs act both on the CTZ and within the GI tract. Several different drugs exist in this class, but the most common you are likely to see and use is ondansetron. This group of drugs is generally considered to be safe and effective and is suitable in a wide range of situations. Occasionally, prolongation of the QT interval may occur – concomitant use of drugs that also prolong the QT interval should be avoided.

Ondansetron 4–8mg, TDS 6°, IV/IM/PO

Other anti-emetics

Other drugs you may occasionally come across for the management of nausea and vomiting include:

1. **Dexamethasone:** Often given in theatre during a general anaesthetic.
2. **Haloperidol:** Used primarily as an antipsychotic/sedative, but also for its anti-emetic properties
3. **Nabilone:** Used occasionally in cases of refractory nausea and vomiting.

---

* The MHRA (Medicines and Healthcare Products Regulatory Agency) has released new guidelines that metoclopramide and domperidone should only be used for the shortest durations possible (for metoclopramide this is for a maximum of 5 days and for domperidone this is for a maximum of 1 week) due to adverse effects.

Intravenous fluids support the cardiovascular system and allow the provision of electrolytes.

They are delivered to patients in the following situations:

1. Patients who are nil by mouth (NBM) and requiring 'maintenance fluid'.
2. Patients who are hypovolaemic from blood loss, dehydration, or sepsis.

Fluids can be subcategorized into crystalloids and colloids.

Colloids

These consist of water to which a substance of high molecular weight is added (e.g. gelatins, dextrans, or starches). Examples you are likely to come across include Gelofusin®, Voluven®, Volplex® and Volulyte®. Due to their high molecular weight, colloids are held within the intravascular space longer than other types of IV fluid. For this reason, they are particularly indicated in situations where the patient is hypovolaemic, i.e. major haemorrhage. Historically, colloids have also been the initial fluid of choice for patients with sepsis. However, recent evidence now suggests that crystalloids are the more favourable fluid in this context.

Crystalloids

These fluids consist of water with the addition of solutes such as glucose and sodium chloride. They provide the mainstay of intravascular fluid therapy and are the most frequently used on general hospital wards. The three most commonly encountered are:

- 0.9% 'normal' saline: 1L = 154mmol of Na^+ and CL^-.
- 5% dextrose: 1L = 278mmol of glucose.
- Hartmann's: 1L = 131mmol Na^+, 5.4mmol K^+, 112mmol CL^-, 29mmol HCO_3^-, 1.8mmol Ca.

As the above demonstrates, Hartmann's provides the most physiological solution. It also contains a lower concentration of chloride, and thus the incidence of hyperchloraemic acidosis (a recognized side effect of large volumes of 0.9% saline) is reduced.

Prescribing maintenance fluid

Maintenance fluid is delivered to patients who are either nil by mouth or unable to take sufficient fluid orally for whatever reason. Maintenance fluid aims to provide the patient's daily requirement of water and electrolytes. In theory, over a 24-hour period, the average euvolaemic patient requires:

- 1–1.5ml/kg/hour of water (2–3L/day).
- 100–150mmol of Na^+.
- 40mmol of K^+.

Therefore, the starting point for a maintenance fluid prescription could be:

- BAG 1: 0.9% saline or Hartmann's over 8 hours.
- BAG 2: 5% dextrose + 20mmol KCL over 8 hours.
- BAG 3: 5% dextrose + 20mmol KCL over 8 hours.

Always check urea and electrolytes (U&E) prior to commencing IV fluid, and make any alterations to the above prescription as necessary. For example, if the patient is:

- Hyponatramic – give more saline/Hartmann's.
- Hypernatraemic – give more 5% dextrose.

Apply the same logic for potassium. If the U&E demonstrates an imbalance, prescribe less or more as indicated.
If a patient does have abnormal baseline electrolytes, try and establish why this is the case and alert a senior if the abnormalities are particularly abnormal.

Giving a fluid challenge

Patients with low BP or oliguria are usually considered for a fluid challenge.
This involves delivering a rapid fluid bolus to a patient followed by an assessment for response. The volume chosen will depend upon the degree of instability but will typically be either 250 or 500ml. The ideal fluid for this is debatable. In reality, either Hartman's solution or normal saline are generally used, whereas 5% dextrose is avoided.
A fluid challenge may be given using a volumetric pump (used on most general wards) or via a giving set with a

three-way tap attached. The method chosen will depend largely on the equipment available in your clinical area.

British Thoracic Society. 2008. Guideline for emergency oxygen use in adult patients. BR O'Driscall, LS Howard, AG Davison. http://www.brit-thoracic.org.uk/document-library/clinical-information/oxygen/emergency-oxygen-use-in-adult-patients

Burdett, Stephen. 2006. 'Blood transfusion: a practical guide'. British Journal of Hospital Medicine. Vol 67, No4.

Clinical Resource Efficiency Support team. 2005. McVeigh, Fitzpatrick, Maxwell, Trinick. 'Guidelines for the treatment if hyperkalaemia in adults. http://www.dhsspsni.gov.uk/hyperkalaemia-booklet.pdf

National Institute of Clinical Excellence. 2008. Diagnosis of acute stroke and transient ischaemic attack (TIA). http://www.nice.org.uk/cg68

National Institute of Clinical Excellence. 2012. Acute upper gastrointestinal bleed management. http://guidance.nice.org.uk/cg141

National Institute of Clinical Excellence. 2013. Acute kidney injury. http://guidance.nice.org.uk/cg169

Survive Sepsis Group. 2012. 'The sepsis six'. http://www.survivesepsis.org

A